The Eight-Step Approach for Student Clinical Success

TOOLS FOR STUDENTS

Lydia R. Zager, MSN, RN
Clinical Professor
Medical/Surgical Nursing
    Coordinator,
College of Nursing,
University of South Carolina
Columbia, South Carolina

JoAnne Herman, PhD, RN
Assistant Dean for Graduate
    Studies
Associate Professor
College of Nursing,
University of South Carolina
Columbia, South Carolina

Loretta Manning, MSN, RN, GNP
President,
I CAN Publishing®, Inc.
Regional Director,
Sylvia Rayfield & Associates
Duluth, Georgia

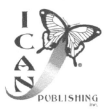

I CAN Publishing®, Inc. ◆ Duluth, GA
www.icanpublishing.com

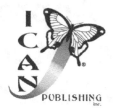

I CAN Publishing®, Inc.
2650 Chattahoochee Drive, Suite 100
Duluth, GA 30097
www.icanpublishing.com

ISBN: 978-0-9842040-5-2
Library of Congress Control Number: 2011924511
Printed in the United States of America
First Edition

Copies of this book may be obtained from:
I CAN Publishing®, Inc.
2650 Chattahoochee Drive, Suite 100
Duluth, GA 30097
1-866-428-5589
www.icanpublishing.com

Cover and interior design by Mary Jo Zazueta/www.tothepointsolutions.com

Contents

About the Authors

DR. JOANNE HERMAN received her PhD in nursing from the University of Texas at Austin. One of her major scholarship activities has been clinical reasoning. She provided leadership in a curriculum revision at the University of South Carolina College of Nursing in 1985 that resulted in the addition of two courses in clinical reasoning. She taught the senior level baccalaureate course for 10 years. In 1995, the curriculum was revised again and she taught the junior level clinical reasoning course. JoAnne was awarded the prestigious Michael. J. Mungo award for undergraduate teaching at the University of South Carolina. She is a known national and international speaker and has been a frequent presenter at many nursing conferences. She is the co-author of *Clinical Reasoning: The Art and Science of Critical and Creative Thinking*. She has multiple publications both theoretical and clinical application related to clinical reasoning. She has served as a consultant for soft ware companies who wanted to include clinical reasoning as the basis for their content presentations.

LORETTA S. MANNING received her MSN from Indiana University and her BSN from Indiana State University. She received her Gerontological Nurse Practitioner certificate from the University of North Carolina in Greensboro, North Carolina. After working as an intensive critical care and charge nurse in pediatric nursing, she became a clinical educator at the University of Indianapolis. In 1984, she taught in the BSN program at Northwestern State University, in Shreveport, Louisiana. Loretta has co-authored *Nursing Made Insanely Easy*, *Pharmacology Made Insanely Easy*, *NCLEX-RN® 101: How to Pass*, and *Pathways of Teaching Nursing: Keeping it Real*. Loretta is a 2004 graduate fellow of the Amy V. Cockcroft Leadership Development Program. She has consulted with schools nationally and internationally in assisting faculty with teaching strategies, for making learning fun and assisting with clinical decision making. Loretta's expertise is in developing faculty and clinical adjunct instructors in the area of connecting NCLEX®, Patient Safety, and Joint Commission Standards both in the classroom as well as in clinical education. She is a Regional Director with Sylvia Rayfield & Associates and leads NCLEX-RN® and Pharmacology NCLEX® review courses across the country. She has one chapter on preparing students for the NCLEX-RN® published in 2008 in the book, *Mastering the Teaching Role: A Guide for Nurse Educators*. She has recently co-developed a medical surgical concept curriculum. Loretta Manning is the President and Co-Founder of I CAN Publishing®, Inc., a company dedicated to improving health care and inspiring educators and learners by transforming education through creating resources to make teaching and learning easy and fun.

LYDIA R. ZAGER earned her MSN in nursing administration with a minor in education at the University of Texas in San Antonio, Texas and her BSN from Pittsburg State University in Pittsburg, Kansas. She is currently a clinical professor in the College of Nursing at the University of South Carolina since 1998. Prior to that, she was a clinical faculty for Central Carolina Technical College. Lydia is a retired Lieutenant Colonel from the Army Nurse Corps and served in a variety of leadership positions in the military to include clinical management, staff advisor, recruitment and chief of hospital education. Lydia is a 2004 graduate fellow of the Amy V. Cockcroft Leadership Development Program. Lydia has gained national and state recognition in clinical nursing education through her consulting, presentations and faculty development workshops. Her expertise is in developing clinical and adjunct nursing instructors particularly in the area of clinical reasoning and organizing the clinical day to help meet patient safety, NCLEX® and Joint Commission Standards. In addition she has years of experience in teaching preceptor workshops and facilitating preceptor programs. She has two chapters on leadership and the multigenerational student published in 2008 in the book, *Mastering the Teaching Role: A Guide for Nurse Educator* and is the co-author of two articles on leadership. She has recently co-developed a medical surgical concept curriculum.

Contributors

Ellen S. Adkins, BSN, RN
Graduate Teaching Assistant
Family Nurse Practitioner (FNP)/
    Doctorate of Nursing Practice (DNP)
    Graduate Student
University of South Carolina
    College of Nursing
Columbia, South Carolina

Kate K. Chappell, MSN, APRN, CPNP
Clinical Assistant Professor
University of South Carolina
    College of Nursing
Columbia, South Carolina

Kimberly Glenn, MN, RN, CPN
Clinical Associate Professor
University of South Carolina
Columbia, South Carolina

Erin M. McKinney, MN, RNC
Clinical Assistant Professor, Director
    Clinical Simulation Laboratory
University of South Carolina
    College of Nursing
Columbia, South Carolina

Jada C. Quinn, DNP, APRN, FNP-BC,
    ACNP-BC
Clinical Assistant Professor
University of South Carolina
Columbia, South Carolina

Sylvia Rayfield, MN, RN, CNS
Board Chairwoman
Sylvia Rayfield & Associates
Dahlonega, Georgia

Ellen C. Synovec, RN, MN, MBA, NEA-BC
Assistant Clinical Professor
University of South Carolina
Columbia, South Carolina

Lisa T. Williams DNP, MSN/Ed., APRN,
    FNP-BC
Clinical Assistant Professor
University of South Carolina
Columbia, South Carolina

Preface

"The most important thing in nursing is not so much to gain more and more facts as to TRANSFORM the way we think about these facts."

~ Loretta Manning, President, I CAN Publishing®, Inc.

Effective clinical education is imperative for the success of nursing education programs, student success as well as outcomes for quality patient care. Nursing programs are expected to develop proficient clinicians upon graduation. This mandates that nursing programs provide excellent clinical experiences where students learn to integrate the theory with competent clinical skills in the care of clients.

During our conversations with nursing students, we were routinely requested to provide a document including all of the clinical teaching tools that were discussed and reviewed. Students requested these tools to assist them in linking theory with clinical decision-making to facilitate both clinical and exam success. They have also requested these tools to simplify the planning process during clinical rotations.

We began the journey to write this book because of the numerous requests from clinical students. We realized this book needed to have a practical approach to clinical learning. We want to provide you with the tools and strategies of how to begin clinical nursing day one and proceed to the last day and final clinical evaluations. Rarely do nursing students get any formal preparation in the area for clinical experiences. There was no road map or compass to guide you through the maze. Since clinical plays a pivotal role in connecting theory to practice, it is imperative to assist you in your vital role to maximize your learning in clinical.

This book contains many tools and forms that can be used as templates in clinical. The tools and information included in this book have been developed from our 38 years of combined clinical experience teaching nursing students in academic settings and nurses in a variety of clinical units from across the country.

We hope this book will be a practical guide for you as you prepare for clinicals. The book is now in your hands to reach your destination.

The Eight-Step Approach for Student Clinical Success is illustrated by using the word **CLINICAL** as indicated below:

C   Clinical: How Do I Start?

L   Learn How to Structure the Clinical Day

I   Improve My Critical Thinking and Clinical Judgment

N   Nursing Concept Map

I   Interactive Strategies for Clinical Learning

C   Collaborating with Multi-Generational Learners

A   Assessment and Evaluation

L   Linking Clinical Experience to NCLEX® Success

There are two ways you can approach this book. Our first recommendation is to read the book in its entirety for continuity of content and a complete picture of the clinical experience. Another approach to expedite your learning or for a refresher, you can refer directly to the area where you need assistance. We hope this book will facilitate your transition into clinical and make this a positive experience. We hope the clinical tools will continue to assist you in guiding your success both on the NCLEX® and in clinical practice and will be a resource to you while you are in school.

We dedicate this work to the many nursing students who are constantly striving for an increased level of excellence.

Acknowledgments

We want to acknowledge and express our appreciation to the clinical faculty at the University of South Carolina in Columbia, South Carolina. We appreciate your contributions, your helpful suggestions, the adaptation and use of many of the forms in this book throughout the clinical courses.

We also want to thank the nursing students across the country and from the University of South Carolina for all of the useful feedback that has assisted us throughout the development of the tools and book.

We want to express our appreciation to each of our family members for their never-ending support and love while we developed this book.

We want to thank Jennifer Robinson, our Administrative Director, who supports us with all aspects of writing, publishing, and distributing our books. We most want to thank her for her love and great sense of humor that keeps us smiling and laughing during the moments we are working to meet deadlines!

The Eight-Step Approach for Student Clinical Success

CHAPTER 1

Clinical Learning: How Do I Start?

IN THIS CHAPTER YOU WILL:

→ Assess your readiness to be a successful student

→ Discover how you as a novice student think and learn

→ Explore the characteristics of novice student learners

ASSESS YOUR READINESS TO BE A CLINICAL NURSING STUDENT

As a clinical nursing student, you are preparing for your important new role as a registered nurse. Through a collaborative partnership with your clinical instructor, you can make learning a positive experience that will set the tone for how you approach client care.

Clinical can be a scary process, but not when you are adequately prepared. Through adequate preparation, clinical is extremely rewarding. This chapter will help you assess your readiness for your clinical experience. The **Clinical Self-Assessment Questionnaire** found at the end of this chapter will help you with this process as you begin your role. If the answer to any of the following questions is "No," the resource column will help you find the information you need.

DISCOVER HOW YOU AS A NOVICE STUDENT THINK AND LEARN

The brain is structured in neural-networks. These networks are established through learning and experience, which is why clinical is so important in the development of a new nurse. We used to believe, for example, that how we baked a cake was all located in one part of the brain. Now we know through fMRI imaging that the knowledge about how to bake a cake is stored all over the brain. The knowledge about how to bake the cake is accessed as we develop neural-networks with increasing numbers of inter-connections through our experience in baking a cake. The more times we bake the cake, the more inter-connections are established, and the more expertise we develop.

That is why experienced nurses are able to reach clinical decisions very quickly. They have an almost infinite number of inter-connections with stored knowledge because of their extensive experience. You, as a novice learner, have minimal inter-connections.

Initial learning is temporary. Repetition is critical for students to learn. The neural-networks become better connected through increased repetition. For example, every time you insert a foley catheter, the relationship among the steps of the procedure, sterile technique, rationale for the foley, potential complications and needed patient teaching increases the strength of the connection of these parts to each other resulting in an increased competence.

EXPLORE THE CHARACTERISTICS OF NOVICE STUDENT LEARNERS

+ They make decisions quickly before thinking about all the options that are possible, in other words, they will jump to conclusions.

+ They have difficulty applying classroom content to clinical situations.

+ They are easily overwhelmed by data, i.e., information in the medical record.

+ They have difficulty distinguishing relevant from irrelevant information.

+ They have low tolerance for ambiguity.

+ They may be unwilling to engage in challenging problems.

+ They want to rely heavily on known solutions.

+ They often have a non-systematic approach to clinical problems.

In addition, novice student learners approach clinical situations in a very apprehensive way. They see clinical as a set of tasks that must be accomplished. Each clinical day is a test of their personal capabilities.

No wonder you feel stressed!! The following chapters provide strategies that you can use to help you progress and give you the tools necessary to be an even better clinical student.

CLINICAL SELF-ASSESSMENT QUESTIONNAIRE

Self-Assessment Questions	Yes, I Know	No, I Need Help	Resources: Where to Find Help
1. Do I understand the expected outcomes of this clinical?			Refer to course syllabus and course coordinator.
2. Do I have the knowledge, skills and abilities to provide safe and effective care?			1. Refer to course text books. 2. Reflect on prior clinical experiences with similar types of clients. 3. Work with other students in your clinical group.
3. In orientation to clinical did I learn: policies and procedures, and medication protocols, documentation, supply systems, safety or quality assurance concerns.			1. Review unit and clinical facilities' policies and procedures. 2. Learn the medication system for the unit, the documentation process, and supply systems.
4. Do I know what the clinical setting offers as learning opportunities?			1. Meet with clinical instructor to discuss learning opportunities available in this clinical unit.. 2. Meet with other members of the interdisciplinary team for the unit.
5. Do I know how to prepare for my clinical experience?			Refer to Chapter 2

6. Do I know how to structure my clinical day? This should include:
  a. orientation to the unit
  b. the clinical day routine
  c. documentation
  d. administer medications
  e. written plans for care
  f. pre and post conference
			Read Chapter 2

7. Do I know what thinking strategies I can use to improve my clinical reasoning?			Chapter 1, 2, 3
8. Do I know how to use NCLEX® activities to organize my learning?			Refer to chapter 8

Handout 1

CLINICAL SELF-ASSESSMENT QUESTIONNAIRE (cont'd)

Self-Assessment Questions	Yes, I Know	No, I Need Help	Resources: Where to Find Help
9. Do I know how to answer inquiry and reflections questions?			Refer to Chapter 3
10. Do I know how to use a concept map in clinical?			Refer to Chapter 4
11. Do I know how to make clinical judgments through the use of thinking strategies?			Refer to Chapter 3
12. Do I know how to use innovative learning strategies in clinical?			Refer to Chapter 5
13. Do I know how to receive formal and informal feedback?			Refer to Chapter 7
14. Do I know how counseling will be used to help me improve my clinical practice and to notify me if I am not meeting clinical requirements?			Refer to Chapter 7
15. Do I know the evaluation outcome criteria that will be used for my clinical performance?			Refer to Chapter 7

CHAPTER 2

Learn How to Structure the Clinical Day

IN THIS CHAPTER YOU WILL LEARN HOW TO:

→ Structure the clinical day

→ Structure medication administration

→ Structure how to organize clinical data

STRUCTURING THE CLINICAL DAY

Many new clinical nursing students feel overwhelmed with how to organize a clinical day. The thought of administering multiple medications alone can result in a sleepless night. Our goal is to provide you with tools and structure to assist you in planning and organizing the clinical day.

Good communication with the staff can make all the difference in the quality of the clinical experience and the relationships among the staff, you, and the clinical instructor. Discuss with your clinical instructor the skills and procedures you can do alone, with the nursing staff, or your clinical instructor. Determine how you will communicate. Coordinate with the staff your clinical assignment and aspects of the care you will be performing.

The next step is to plan your clinical day. The first chart provides an example of how to structure a typical clinical day. The structure will decrease your anxiety and optimize your learning experience. The chart **How to Structure a Typical Clinical Day**, found at the end of the chapter, can be adapted to your clinical setting. It may seem like a lot of work, but the time spent in planning will help ensure your success.

STRUCTURING MEDICATION ADMINISTRATION

The second chart found at the end of the chapter is a **Medication Protocol: A Fail Safe Approach**. It is imperative that students master a structure to develop safe medication administration practices. When students consistently use a structured process, you develop safe medication administration habits essential to prevent medication errors. The medication protocol not only helps you administer medications safely and efficiently, but it also helps you feel confident that you are prepared to give your medications.

In order for the medication protocol to have the maximum effect, you need to use it throughout all of your clinical courses. This prevents you from having to learn a new structure for giving medications with each clinical instructor. This consistency throughout the courses provides repetition and strengthens the safe medication administration habit.

STRUCTURING HOW TO ORGANIZE CLINICAL DATA

Students are overwhelmed with how to organize the information you get from report and orders for procedures and medications. Without a structured format, you are disorganized in thinking, delivery of care, and timeliness. This disorganization makes it difficult for you to document accurately. At the end of the chapter is an example of a **Student Report Sheet** that you can use when receiving report at the beginning of clinical.

Also included at the end of the chapter are examples of a Typical Day Events and a description of a Shift Report Using SBAR Format. We have found these two handouts to be extremely useful to help you organize your day and learn how to give an effective and accurate report using SBAR. The tools help you understand the expectations for clinical performance, document with accuracy, and most importantly, provide safe and effective care in a timely manner.

HOW TO STRUCTURE A TYPICAL CLINICAL DAY

Time	Student Activity	How Your Clinical Instructor May Help You (The following are examples.)
6:45 AM When you arrive for clinical prior to pre-conference time . . .	Get report (SBAR) from your nurse. Check for: • New orders • New medications • Time of 1st medication • Check if NPO for tests, surgery or procedures. If so, will they get any of their meds, i.e., insulin, antihypertensives?	The goal for clinical faculty prior to the beginning of clinical is to determine: • What student, what client, what skills, what medications are going to require your attention? • How will you prioritize and guide the students in prioritizing their activities? Example: • Prioritize the student's learning needs (i.e., Trach suctioning and does the student have the skill?) • Prioritize assigned client's needs (i.e., acuity, medications times; i.e., 7 AM medication) • Know what diagnostic exams (i.e., are they NPO for cardiac cath?)
Pre-conference	Share clinical concept maps and plans for the day	Assess if the students are prepared: • Do they have their clinical concept map with predicted client's needs and interventions and are they accurate? • Use inquiry questions in your assessment • Schedule student activities that require clinical instructor supervision beginning with early AM medications and scheduled procedures
7:00 – 7:20 AM	See your client for a quick assessment: • Respiratory status, in pain, safety issues, etc. • Check IVs. Make sure they are patent and running at the right rate with the right fluid • Check for any other lines, tubes, that they are patent, and note the drainage • Take B/P and pulse • Check on blood sugars or obtain glucometer reading • Administer insulin or other before meals medications • (Always check to see if the med has been given, is being held, etc.) • Prepare for any scheduled tests	• Use Medication protocol • Meet students as scheduled

HOW TO STRUCTURE A TYPICAL CLINICAL DAY (cont'd)

Time	Student Activity	How Your Clinical Instructor May Help You (The following are examples.)
8:00 – 9:30 AM	• Give AM medications • Perform other client procedures as ordered • Prepare client for scheduled procedures/surgery if scheduled • Complete physical assessment • Complete or ensure AM care is done (often a good time to assess and do your physical)	• Use medication protocol • Divide students into groups • Have part of the students begin with medication administration • Have part of the students complete AM care and do assessments • Recommend doing procedures that require supervision after AM medications are given
9:30 – 10 AM	• First documentation entered to include assessments and other findings • Implement and evaluate your nursing interventions, i.e., coughing and deep breathing • Turn or ambulate your client • Assess activity tolerance	Begin making rounds of student's clients: • See priority clients first, i.e. and indwelling lines, IVs, tubes, unstable clients • Facilitate students with their care • Ask students inquiry questions &/or reflection questions (see chart in Chapter 3 for suggestions)
10:30 AM	• Continue to assess client and document • Evaluate response to PRN medications • Complete any treatments or procedures as ordered (This may be earlier depending on the time of the test) • Client teaching and documentation • Continue to check for new doctor's orders • Check for lab result, i.e., PTT if on heparin	• Ensure students have completed assessments, evaluations and documents of client's progress toward outcomes • Assist students with other procedures, changes in doctors' orders as needed, etc.
11:00 – 12:00	• Give medications as ordered • Feed patient • Assess vital signs as ordered • Continue to assess client and document findings • Care for indwelling lines • Continue interventions and assess effectiveness	Assist students as needed

HOW TO STRUCTURE A TYPICAL CLINICAL DAY (cont'd)

Time	Student Activity	How Your Clinical Instructor May Help You (The following are examples.)
Lunch	• Plan your lunch around your client's needs (you will need to cover for your fellow students)	• Schedule student and your breaks and meals around client's needs • Depending on the level of the students, i.e. if this is their first semester versus a senior nursing student, decide if they will cover for each other or go as a group
1:00 – 1:45 PM	• Continue to assess if client outcomes are being met and document • Continue client teaching and document • Complete any scheduled interventions or procedures	• Continue rounds of students' clients • Ensure students have completed their care
1:45 – 2:30 PM	• Complete final assessment and document client's progress toward outcomes • Document I & O • Record IV and other drainage • Make sure client is safe • Room is neat • Check to see if all medications have been given and documented with client responses	• Evaluate student documentation • Has the student documented the client's response to interventions and progress toward outcomes? • Do their notes include changes in the client's assessment? • Are I & O's recorded? • Are there any medications, treatments or procedures that have not been done? • Make quick rounds to ensure all patients are safe
2:30 PM	Give SBAR to the assigned nurse	Ensure all students have reported off using SBAR to the assigned nurse
2:30 – 3:00 PM	Post conference	Conduct post conference using inquiry and reflection questions (see charts in Chapter 3 for examples)
	Go home and be thankful another clinical day is over and you are one day closer to graduation! Seriously, spend some time reflecting over your experience and answer assigned reflections questions.	Take time to reflect on how the day went and what you can do to improve the next clinical day with your students.

MEDICATION PROTOCOL: A FAIL SAFE APPROACH

1. Prior to beginning medication administration:
   a. Verify orders
   b. Gather needed client assessments (i.e., B/P, pulse, or other required assessment data)
   c. Check needed lab results (i.e., potassium level if client has lasix ordered, blood sugar or glucometer readings for insulin, drug levels)
   d. Check to see if any clients are NPO, or are going for procedures, dialysis, etc.

2. Pull the Medication Record for your client (the MAR). Do only one client at a time.
3. Obtain the medications you need (your clinical instructor may have to do this for you based on the medication system in your facility, i.e., scanners).
4. Lay your MAR on the counter and/or use the computer screen to check your medications, vials, IV piggy backs, IV fluids beside the name on the sheet.

5. Know what each of your medications is: Do you have all the information you need prior to giving the medication? If not, obtain and review this information and have it ready.
   a. Action
   b. Key side effects
   c. Nursing implications
   d. Why the client is getting the medication?
   e. Food/drug or drug/drug interactions
   f. Known allergies
   g. What do you need to teach your patient about the medication?

6. Check the medications against the MAR in order as they are listed to ensure: (leave medications in their wrappers and do not draw medications from the vials without your clinical instructor).
   a. Do you have the right medication?
   b. Is the medication scheduled at this time?
   c. Is it the right dose?
   d. Is there any information you need prior to giving the medication, i.e., B/P readings, digoxin levels you do not have?
   e. Has the medication already been given?
   f. Based on what you know about the medication, does it make sense (rationale) that this client would be getting this medication?
   g. Is there any information that needs to be recorded on the MAR prior to giving the medication, i.e., blood pressure?

7. Let your instructor know you are ready to check off your medications.
8. Go through information listed in Step number 5 with your clinical instructor. At this time, adjust any dosages, i.e., cut the pill, pull up the correct dose for injections.
9. Once you have completed the check-off with your faculty, take your MAR and the medications still in their wrappers (or the scanner) to the client's bedside.
10. Perform seven rights for medications, check your meds as you open them with the MAR.
11. Sign off the medications on the MAR as the client takes them and perform necessary client teaching.
12. Return the MAR to the appropriate place or scanner and note when your next medications are due. Document client teaching.
13. Evaluate client's response to medications.
14. Document client's response and progress toward outcome.

STUDENT REPORT SHEET

0700	0800	0900	1000
Client Initials	Check BS ___	Med Administration	Hourly Rounding
Room	24 hour BS trends ___	Rhythm ___ Rate ___	Chart: Client activity
Safety Huddle	Give Insulin	Begin Treatments	Treatments
AM Report	Breakfast	Clinical Paperwork	Ambulate
System Review	Hourly Rounding		Rhythm ___ Rate ___
Check line patency**	Chart: Client activity		Clinical Paperwork
List treatments needed	Client Education		
SBAR	Med Administration		
*Always review and note trends!	Rhythm ___ Rate ___		
LABS :			
I&Os:			
VS: T° ___ BP ___ HR ___ RR ___			
Sat % ___			
Man: BP ___ HR ___ RR ___			
VS: 24 hour trends:			

1100	1200	1300	1400
Eat Lunch	Check BS ___	Wrap Up:	Report off: SBAR
Treatments	Give Insulin	Treatments	Post-conference Points
Ambulate	Lunch ___	Clinical Paperwork	
Rhythm ___ Rate ___	Hourly Rounding	Chart: I & O	
Clinical Paperwork	Chart: Client activity	*Clear Pumps	
	Rhythm ___ Rate ___	Rhythm ___ Rate ___	
		Give 1400 meds if assigned	
	VS: T° ___ BP ___ HR ___ RR ___	Review Charting	
	Sat ___		
	Man: BP ___ HR ___ RR ___		
	*Indicate Normal/Abnormal and Report		

TYPICAL DAY EVENTS
(May vary per clinical and patient needs)

When you arrive, before 6:45 AM
+ Get report from your nurse
+ Check for new orders, new meds, time of first med, check if NPO for test, which meds are they getting, AM blood sugars

7:00 – 7:20 AM Preconference
+ Take B/P and pulse
+ Give 7:30 meds, insulin (check to see if it has been given)
+ See your pt, assess quickly, check IVs, make sure they are patent and running at the right rate with the right fluid, check for any other lines, tubes that they are patent and what is draining

By 9:30 AM
+ Give meds and complete assessment or vise versa as appropriate
+ Give assessment to your nurse to enter in the computer
+ AM care (you may do part of your assessment then)

10 AM
+ Chart opening nursing note with AM assessment by_____(Time)

10:30 AM
+ Treatments or procedures ordered (This may come earlier if scheduled for tests.)
+ Do patient teaching as needed. Continue to check for new Dr.'s orders
+ Check for lab results, particularly PTT if on heparin. 11:00–12:00 check for noon BS if ordered, eat lunch, feed pt if needed

11 AM
+ Vital signs (give results to techs) Continue to assess patient's response and progress toward outcomes.

Lunch for 30 min between the hours of 11:00 and 12:00 based on your patient's needs and schedules

Give 11 and 12 o'clock meds if ordered, Flush INTs
+ Continue to reinforce patient teaching and interventions to help your patients achieve the outcomes and continuously reassess your patient

1:00 PM
+ Wrap-up, do final assessment, make sure patient is okay and room is neat
+ Do I & O and chart results. Check to see if all meds have been given and charted.

1:30 PM
+ Chart final notes: include evaluation of your patient's progress or lack of progress toward the outcomes. How is he doing? Is he getting better? Include I & O and record again information on IVs, drains, etc.

By 2:00 PM
+ Report off to your nurse and your clinical instructor using SBAR

2:00 PM Post-conference

SHIFT REPORT USING SBAR FORMAT

The Situation and Background will only need to be entered the first time you report on this client.

Situation: Patient Name, Age, Sex

Room Number

Physician(s)

Background: Admission Diagnosis (date of surgery)

Past medical history that is significant (hypertension, CHF, etc)

Allergies

This information should be included in each report if applicable.

Assessment: Code Status (any advance directives, DNR orders, POAHC)

Procedures done in previous 24 hours including results/outcomes (include where we stand with post procedure vitals/assessment)

Abnormal assessment findings

Abnormal vital signs

IV fluids/drips/site; when is site to be changed

Current pain score—what has been done to manage pain

Safety Needs—fall risk, skin risk, etc.

Recommendations: Needed changes in the plan of care (diet, activity, medication, consultations)?

What are you concerned about?

Discharge planning

Pending labs/x-rays, etc

Calls out to Dr. _____ about_____

What the next shift needs to do or be aware of—i.e., labs to be drawn in AM

NOTES

CHAPTER 3

Improving Critical Thinking and Clinical Judgment

IN THIS CHAPTER YOU WILL LEARN HOW TO:

→ Develop inquiry questions

→ Develop reflection questions

→ Apply inquiry and reflection questions

→ Use thinking strategies to develop clinical judgment

Now that you have a structure for organizing your clinical day, a protocol for medication administration, and a tool to help you organize your care, it is time to help you improve your critical thinking and clinical judgment skills. When we have worked with clinical facilities, they want their new graduate nurses to have critical thinking skills. Observation of student performance is a part of your clinical instructor's role. However, observation does not give your clinical instructor information on what you are thinking. When your clinical instructor observes you and asks questions in a deliberate and systematic way, it strengthens your critical thinking skills. We have developed two methods of questioning to help you acquire critical thinking skills and improve your ability to make clinical judgments.

DEVELOP INQUIRY QUESTIONS

Inquiry questions require the students to reveal what you know. There is a hierarchy of inquiry questions from knowledge to synthesis. It is essential for clinical instructors to ask you questions that take you beyond memorization of facts to application, analysis, and synthesis. The chart below gives examples of questions that help take you from basic facts to clinical judgment. Asking inquiry questions helps your clinical instructors determine if the you know how to give safe and effective care. This also helps you learn the kind of questions you need to ask yourself when the clinical instructor is not present. Your clinical instructor may begin the inquiry process with knowledge level questions:

✦ Do you know the basic facts?

✦ If you know facts, apply the facts to the total client's care.

✦ If you can apply the facts to the care, review with your instructor the appropriate choices among the options.

✦ If these options are successful, review questions that require you to consider knowledge, past experience and the client's situation simultaneously needed to make clinical judgments.

The table below gives examples of each of these types of questions.

Types of Inquiry Questions

DEFINITIONS	EXAMPLES OF INQUIRY QUESTIONS
Knowledge: Memorized information /facts	What is the normal range for blood pressure?
Application: Connecting knowledge to a clinical situation	Which is the most important vital sign to monitor in your client who has hypertension?
Analysis: Understanding pros & cons, strengths and weaknesses or options in decision-making	In your client with a blood pressure of 95/60, should you administer the anti-hypertensive medication as ordered?
Synthesis: Pulling together multiple sources of experiences, data and information to make judgments about needed client care. This process may require several inquiry questions to guide the student.	What has the blood pressure been for the past two days? Is this the same or has there been a change? What could be contributing to this change in their B/P? Are there any guidelines in the doctor's orders regarding their B/P? What nursing actions will you take?

At the end of the chapter, **The Quick Approach: Inquiry Questions Organized Around the Nursing Process** will provide you with multiple examples of questions that you can ask yourself in different client care situations.

DEVELOP REFLECTION QUESTIONS

Reflection questions require you to think about your own thinking. Reflection challenges you to self-monitor, plan, and revise your own thinking so you can quickly self-correct. Reflection results in safe and effective decisions about the needed client care and the prevention of complications. Reflective thinking is an essential component of clinical judgment. Included at the end of the chapter in handout 2 is an **Example of Reflection Questions** that you can use to reflect on your clinical experience for the day. You may be asked to share your reflections in a post conference. This example includes points that are a part of the **Criteria for the Outcome Web** (Chapter 4, handout 2). Reflection questions can be changed weekly and adapted to meet the needs of the clinical day. The mark of a true professional is to reflect constantly about their clinical practice.

APPLY INQUIRY AND REFLECTION QUESTIONS

At the end of the chapter, handout 3, is a **Urinary Catheterization Algorithm** that displays how your clinical instructor might use inquiry and reflection questions before, during, and after a urinary catherization. The questions included in the algorithm help you see beyond the task to the clinical judgment needed even with procedures. These same types of questions apply to any procedure.

USE THINKING STRATEGIES TO DEVELOP CLINICAL JUDGMENT

Clinical judgment is not inherent in a novice thinker. You can use inquiry and reflection questions to help you adopt a structured way of thinking about a client situation. This process will help you build clinical judgment skills. The chart **Thinking Strategies to Improve Student's Clinical Judgment**, at the end of the chapter, lists thinking strategies, their definitions, and use of them in clinical. The chart combines thinking strategies with inquiry and reflection questions. If you use the thinking strategies in the chart, you will improve your clinical judgment. The chart also describes the purpose and rationale for use by your clinical instructor.

NOTES

THE QUICK APPROACH: INQUIRY QUESTIONS FOR CLINICAL KNOWLEDGE ORGANIZED AROUND THE NURSING PROCESS

Assessment

1. Which vital sign assessments would be the highest priority for a client with a specific clinical diagnosis (i.e., temperature, pulse, respiratory rate, and blood pressure) and why?

2. Which of the above vital signs should be reported to a team member or provider of care and why?

3. Which assessments would be a priority for your client (i.e., BP, bradycardia, bleeding, etc.) and why?

4. What is the highest priority nursing action before initiating an order? (Check/verify accuracy of order)

5. Which assessment finding is a priority for monitoring your client's hydration status (i.e., I & O, edema, signs and symptoms of dehydration)?

6. Which of your clients should be assessed/triaged initially and why?

7. Which of the psychosocial, spiritual, cultural and occupational assessment findings may affect the client's care (i.e., cultural—dietary, occupational—stress, etc.) and why?

Analysis/Diagnosis

1. Prior to administering the medication, which data would be most pertinent to review (i.e., vital signs, lab results, allergies, etc.)?

2. When adjusting or titrating dosage of medications, what physiological parameters did you use (i.e., giving insulin according to blood sugar levels, titrating medication to maintain a specified blood pressure, etc.)?

3. Which systems-specific assessment or reassessments would be the priority for your client and why (i.e., GI, respiratory, cardiac, etc.)?

4. How will you prioritize your care based on the information you received in shift report and why?

5. Which level of nursing personnel would be most appropriate to assign to your client if you were making out assignments (i.e., LPN, VN, assistive personnel, other RNs, etc.)?

6. Which of the clients would be most appropriate to transfer to the (medical surgical unit, orthopedic, psychiatric, etc.) unit?

Outcomes

1. What clinical outcomes best determine the effect of the pain medication?

2. What assessment findings indicate an improvement in the client's hydration status?

3. What clinical findings are expected when the dopamine dosage is titrated appropriately?

4. What clinical findings are expected when the insulin is titrated according to the blood sugar levels?

5. Which assessment findings indicate a positive outcome from the albuterol (Ventolin) treatment?

6. Which assessment findings indicate positive outcomes from (specific medications)?

7. After a specific diagnostic test (i.e., cardiac catheterization, liver biopsy, stress test, etc.), and what clinical outcomes indicate a complication?

THE QUICK APPROACH: INQUIRY QUESTIONS FOR CLINICAL KNOWLEDGE ORGANIZED AROUND THE NURSING PROCESS (cont'd)

Plan

1. Which plan would be most effective for maintaining client confidentiality/privacy?

2. What steps are most important when administering medications by the oral route or gastric tube (i.e., PO, sublingual, nasogastric tube, G tube, etc.)?

3. What plan is most appropriate for preparing medication for administration (i.e., crush medications as needed and appropriate, place in appropriate administrative device, assemble equipment, etc.)?

4. What should be included in the plan to avoid when administering medications (i.e., food, fluids, and other drugs) to minimize medication interactions?

5. What nursing care is important to include in the plan for a client receiving oxygen therapy?

6. What plan is most appropriate when using equipment in performing client care procedures and treatment?

7. What is the priority plan for maintaining your client's skin integrity (i.e., skin care, turn client, etc.)?

8. Which plan would be most appropriate to protect your client from injury (i.e., falls, electrical hazards, malfunctioning equipment, rugs, clutter, etc.)?

9. Which assessment findings would result in the nurse developing a plan to collaborate with other disciplines while providing care to the client (i.e., physician, RT, PT, radiology, dietary, lab, etc.)?

10. What is the plan for assisting the client in the performance of activities of daily living (i.e., ambulation, reposition, hygiene, transfer to chair, eating, toileting, etc.)?

11. What plan is most important to develop after evaluating the risk assessment profile for your client (i.e., sensory impairment, potential for falls, level of mobility, etc.) and why?

12. How does your plan of care address the special needs of the elderly client?

Implement

1. What nursing intervention would have the highest priority for promoting infection control for your client (i.e., hand washing, appropriate room assignment, isolation, aseptic/sterile technique, universal precautions)?

2. Which nursing actions will be most appropriate with medication administration (Implement the Rights of medication administration)?

3. During an IV infusion, what is most important to monitor and maintain (i.e., infusion site, equipment, flushing infusion devices, checking, rates, fluid, and sites, etc.)?

4. What is the priority intervention for your client who is receiving medication by the intravenous route (i.e., IVP, IVPB, PCA pump, continuous infusion fluids, parenteral nutrition) or by SC, IM, intradermal or topical or in the form of eye, ear or nose drops, sprays, ointments or by inhalation (including nebulizer or metered dose inhaler)?

5. Which calculations did you use for medication administration?

6. Which health care provider orders have you received and implemented today and/or transcribed?

7. What regulations did you comply with when working with controlled substances (i.e., counting narcotics, wasting narcotics, etc.)?

8. What information did you share with the client/family regarding the medication regimen, treatments, and/or procedures?

9. Which nursing actions are most important when performing a head-to-toe assessment?

10. How did you perform the health history and how was the information utilized?

THE QUICK APPROACH: INQUIRY QUESTIONS FOR CLINICAL KNOWLEDGE ORGANIZED AROUND THE NURSING PROCESS (cont'd)

11. When communicating with your client, what is your best response?

12. What therapeutic communication techniques were used to support your client or family and/or increase client understanding of his/her behavior?

13. What interventions would be effective in assisting client with emotional and spiritual needs?

14. When performing a diagnostic test (i.e., O_2 saturation, glucose monitoring, testing for occult blood, gastric pH, urine specific gravity, etc.) what are the most important interventions?

15. Which interventions would be the highest priority to manage/prevent possible complications of your client's condition and/or procedure (i.e., circulatory complications, seizures, aspiration, potential neurological complications, etc.) or a client on a ventilator?

16. How did you act as a client advocate during the clinical experience?

17. What intervention was used to provide client and family with information about condition/illness, expected progression, and/or possible outcomes?

18. What procedures did you implement in order to admit, transfer or discharge the client?

19. What steps did you take in discontinuing or removing: IV, NG, urethral catheter, or other lines or tubes?

20. What is the appropriate nursing care for devices and equipment used for drainage (i.e., surgical wound drains, chest tube suction, or drainage devices, urethral catheter care, etc.)?

21. Which nursing intervention would be a priority for providing therapy for comfort and treatment of inflammation, swelling (i.e., apply heat and cold treatments, elevate limb, etc.)?

22. What are the appropriate steps in performing or assisting with a dressing change (i.e., wound, central line dressing, etc.)?

Evaluation

1. Which documentation is most appropriate for a procedure, treatment, or medication and what is the client's response?

2. Is the medication order appropriate for your client (i.e., appropriate for the client's condition, given by appropriate route, in appropriate dosage, etc.)?

3. What documentation in the chart indicates an understanding of the appropriate education necessary for client and family regarding pain management?

4. Which documentation evaluates teaching performed and the level of understanding of client, family or staff?

5. Which documentation indicates the client and family have been educated about his/her rights and responsibilities?

6. Which documentation indicates that the client has given informed consent for treatment?

7. What information in report indicates an understanding of priority information to include for the client(s)?

8. After a specific diagnostic test (i.e., lab, radiology, EKG, etc.), what results would be the most concern for your client?

9. After initiating the plan of care, how did you evaluate the client care (i.e., multidisciplinary care plan, care map, critical pathway, etc.)?

10. Which clinical findings indicate a need to evaluate the client's weight?

EXAMPLE OF REFLECTION QUESTIONS

Student Name _____ Clinical Instructor _____

Sec # _____   Date_____   Sat/UnSat or Grade_____

Due to Clinical Instructor: _____

12 points possible and will be added to Outcome Web Criteria Grading Sheet

1. Explain your rationale for choosing your priority nursing outcomes. (3 points)

2. Describe the relationships and/or rationales for the care, medications and/or treatments ordered and provided for your client today based on the reason for their admission to the hospital. (6 points)

3. What went well today for you in clinical and why? (1 point)

4. What would you do differently if you could and why? (1 point)

5. Today I learned . . . (1 point)

URINARY CATHETERIZATION ALGORITHM

Expected Outcome: Urinary flow established through the catheter while maintaining asepsis and patient comfort.

Inquiry and Reflection Questions about Insertion of a Foley Catheter

Why does this client need a foley? (Application)

Possible answers: Fluid management, incontinence, post-op renal or urinary rocedures

What are potential complications for this client from having a foley? (Application)

Possible answers: Urinary tract infections, skin irritations

What is important to monitor in this client with a foley? (Application)

Possible answers: I & O, signs of infection, color, odor, amount of urine

What are the infection control issues for this client with a foley? (Application)

Possible answers: Sterile procedure, potential UTI from the catheter, obtaining specimens

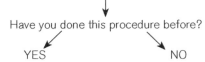

Have you done this procedure before?

YES   NO

What went well with that procedure? (Monitoring)   Name steps of procedure. (Knowledge)
What will you do differently this time? (Revise)   What problems do you anticipate with this
What went wrong with the procedure? (Evaluation)   client? (Application)
How did you problem solve? (Monitoring)   What are possible solutions to these
How will you problem-solve differently this time? (Revise)   potential problems? (Analysis)

Clinical instructors observe the student doing the procedure

Clinical instructor's evaluation of procedure or process

Was the student able to give individualized care with the task?

T –   Techniques of communication with consideration of the individual

A –   Assessment, A & P, Asepsis

S -   Safety

K –   Knowledge and correct implementation of the procedure/skill

YES   NO

Give positive feedback.   Give feedback that the student needs improvement

Document on evaluation form.   Give specific (TASK) feedback to the students on
                                         their performance.
                                       Give them specific behaviors they need to change
                                         before performing a catheterization again.

                                       Evaluate based on previous experience with
                                         catheterizations.

                                       Document on evaluation form.

NOTES

THINKING STRATEGIES TO IMPROVE STUDENT'S CLINICAL JUDGMENT

Thinking Strategies	Definitions	Faculty Strategies	Inquiry Questions Examples	Reflection Questions Examples
Knowledge Work	• Active use of reading, memorizing, drilling, writing, reviewing, and practicing to learn clinical vocabulary and facts.	• Set the structure and expectations required for preparation prior to clinical • Give clear feedback on what knowledge they need to know, i.e., drug-action of medication	• Why does a client with heart failure have edema?	• What knowledge did I need about heart failure that I did not know? • What do I need to know before I care for a heart failure client again?
Prototype Identification	• Using a model case as a reference point for comparative analysis.	• Compare students' clients to prototype in the textbooks or learned in the class room.	• How would a prototype case of congestive heart failure present?	• Were you able to recognize how your client was different from the prototype? • What changes will you make in the care you give next time?
Hypothesizing	• Generating potential options • Recognizing multiple approaches to an outcome or problem	• Have students hypothesize priority nursing diagnosis(es)/problems, assessment data and priority interventions based on their client's medical diagnosis(es) prior to the beginning of clinical using concept mapping or care plans.	• What focused assessment data do you need to confirm or change your diagnosis(es) / problems? • Which of your proposed interventions are applicable? • Do you need to add or change other interventions?	• Was I able to identify the appropriate nursing diagnosis(es)/problems and interventions for my client? • If yes, I confirmed my diagnosis(es)/problems and interventions by_____. • If not, I needed to change, delete or add the following diagnoses/problems and interventions because _____.
Self-Talk	• Expressing one's thoughts to one's self	• Use self-talk (talk aloud to the students as you think about a situation/problem) with the students.	• Talk aloud to me about how you will auscultate your client's lung sounds.	• Was I able to auscultate the lung sounds correctly; and if so, what do the sounds mean related to my care of the client?
Schema Search	• Accessing general/specific patterns of past experiences that might apply to the current case.	• Uses talk aloud method to solicit past clinical experiences.	• How does this congestive heart failure client compare to the heart failure client you took care of last week?	• Based on your experiences with congestive heart failure clients, what patterns of care do you see?

THINKING STRATEGIES TO IMPROVE STUDENT'S CLINICAL JUDGMENT (cont'd)

Thinking Strategies	Definitions	Faculty Strategies	Inquiry Questions Examples	Reflection Questions Examples
If Then Thinking	• Linking ideas and consequences together in a logical sequence	• Ask students questions about potential clinical decisions they could make and what would be the consequences of those decisions.	• If you give the medicine now, what will happen? If you hold the medication, what will happen?	• Did I make the right decision about giving/holding the medication? If not, what would I do differently next time?
Compare & Contrast	• Comparing the strengths and weaknesses of competing alternatives	• Have students identify all the priority interventions with their strengths and weaknesses.	• What would be the most effective intervention(s) to help improve this client's breathing?	• Did I choose the most effective/efficient intervention to improve my client's breathing? • If yes, I knew it was the most effective outcome because … If no, I would do what differently next time?
Trending	• Comparing the client's clinical presentation from one observation to the next observation	• Have students compare, contrast and trend their assessments of their clients they made in the beginning of the clinical with the assessments they make throughout the clinical day.	• What were the trends you identified in the assessments you made of your client? • Are there any changes in your assessment? • What actions do you need to take based on your assessment?	• Was I able to identify the trends and changes accurately? • Were your actions appropriate? • If yes, I knew because…. • If no, I would do what differently?

CHAPTER 4

Nursing Concept Map

IN THIS CHAPTER YOU WILL LEARN HOW TO:

➡ Discuss the advantages of a concept map compared to the traditional care plan

➡ How to construct and use a concept map
  - ◊ Step 1– Begin with the Medical Diagnoses
  - ◊ Step 2 – Generate (hypothesize) the possible client problems/nursing diagnoses
  - ◊ Step 3 – Determine relationships among the client problems/nursing diagnoses
  - ◊ Step 4 – Add clinical assessment findings to the concept map
  - ◊ Step 5 – Determine Outcomes and Evaluation Criteria
  - ◊ Step 6 – Interventions
  - ◊ Step 7 – Evaluation and Clinical Judgment
  - ◊ Step 8 – Documentation

➡ Put the concept map into clinical practice

The concept map provides an excellent tool to help students develop clinical reasoning skills. It is a strategy to externalize thinking, layer levels of clinical reasoning, and promote understanding of interrelationships. It is very typical for novices to focus on one particular assessment, nursing diagnoses or intervention without an understanding of the complexity and interrelationships of the care needed for the client. The concept map helps you see the full scope of the client situation and assists in your thinking about your plan of care. The chart on the next page compares the advantages of using the concept map compared to the traditional five-column care plan in helping you develop clinical reasoning.

ADVANTAGES OF THE CONCEPT MAP
COMPARED TO THE TRADITIONAL CARE PLAN

Concept Map	Traditional Five-Column Care Plan
Visual picture of the interrelationships among the nursing diagnoses /problems	Nursing problems/nursing diagnoses seen in isolation
Systems approach	Linear approach
Outcome thinking	Problem thinking
Focuses on nursing priorities	Focuses on medical/disease
Decision making	Task oriented
Total pages 1–2	Depends on number of nursing diagnoses and can go on and on . . .

The following pages include the step-by-step approach to constructing and using the concept map.

HOW TO CONSTRUCT AND USE A CONCEPT MAP

You begin clinical by receiving your client assignment with the medical diagnoses. The nursing process guides the steps in the development of the concept map.

STEP 1: Place the medical diagnoses/client situation in the middle of the paper with any pertinent client history that would impact the current admission.

Med DX: CHF
Hx: Chronic
Renal Disease

STEP 2: Generate (hypothesize) the possible client problems/nursing diagnoses that might be associated with the medical diagnoses.

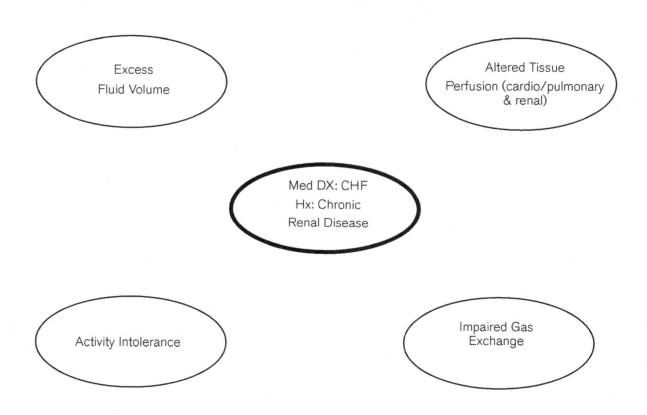

STEP 3: Determine the relationships among the client problems/nursing diagnoses. Here is what you would ask yourself: *"Is there any logical reason why these two problems might be related to each other?"*

a. *"Is there any logical reason why excess fluid volume would be related to activity intolerance?"*

b. If the answer is yes, draw a line to connect them.

c. In this example, excess fluid volume leads to activity intolerance, so draw the line between excess fluid volume and activity intolerance.

d. Working systematically around the circle, you will ask yourself, *"Is excess fluid volume related to the other client's problems/nursing diagnoses included on the map?"*

e. Now ask, *"Is there any logical reason why excess fluid volume is related to impaired gas exchange?"*

f. If the answer is yes, draw a line between the excess fluid volume and impaired gas exchange.

g. In this case, excess fluid volume leads to impaired gas exchange.

h. Finally ask, *"Is there any logical reason why excess fluid volume is related to altered tissue perfusion?"*

i. If the answer is yes, draw the line between excess fluid volume and altered tissue perfusion.

j. In this example, excess fluid volume leads to altered tissue perfusion.

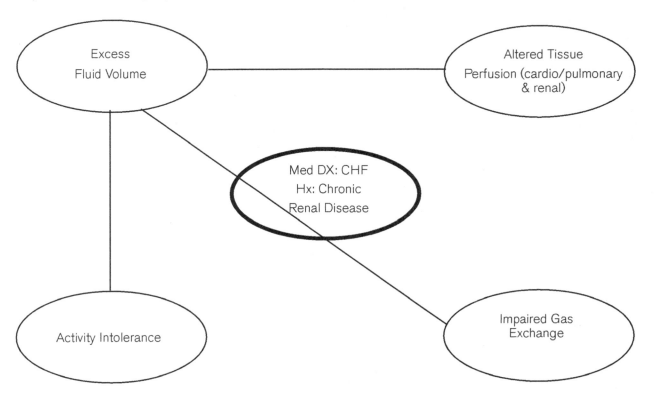

The first layer of the map is complete. We now begin with the next layer of the map.

Repeat the process for all of the nursing diagnoses listed asking the same questions about the relationships between one diagnosis and another. If the answer is yes, draw a line between the two diagnoses.

As you can see, all of these client problems/nursing diagnoses are highly interrelated. So interventions aimed at one client problem/nursing diagnoses may help with the other client problems/nursing diagnoses. The goal is to select priority interventions based on clinical assessment findings that will have the greatest impact on the client's problem.

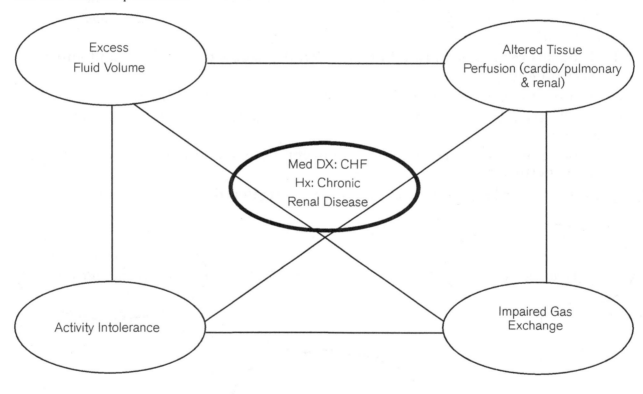

Learning point: It is important for you to determine the priority client problems or needs and what are not. As a student, you often want to include anxiety, risk for infection on every client's concept map because you have learned that these concepts are important for the psychosocial and physiological needs. Yes, it is important for you to assess for anxiety and take steps to prevent infection, but add these to the concept map only if your clinical assessment findings support it.

STEP 4: Add clinical assessment findings to the concept map. The following chart illustrates how assessment data are added to the concept map with the nursing diagnosis of excess fluid volume.

Defining S/SX for Excess Fluid Volume	**Actual** Clinical Assessment Findings
Weight gain >2 lbs. in 24 hours	Weight 120 lbs. yesterday, today 124 lbs.
SOB	SOB
Rales/rhonchi	Yes, R LLobe
Edema	No Edema

Each client's nursing diagnoses chosen by you has a set of defining signs and symptoms that indicate the client nursing diagnoses. You will now complete your assessment of the client and compare their actual assessment clinical findings to the defining signs and symptoms. This comparison will tell you if the client has the nursing diagnosis/problem or not. As students, you normally associate signs and symptoms with something that is wrong. The goal for you is to focus as much attention to positive indicators as well as negative indicators. For example, if you assess for the defining signs and symptoms of excess fluid volume and there is no edema, it is a very important positive assessment clinical finding. It does not mean, however, you stop

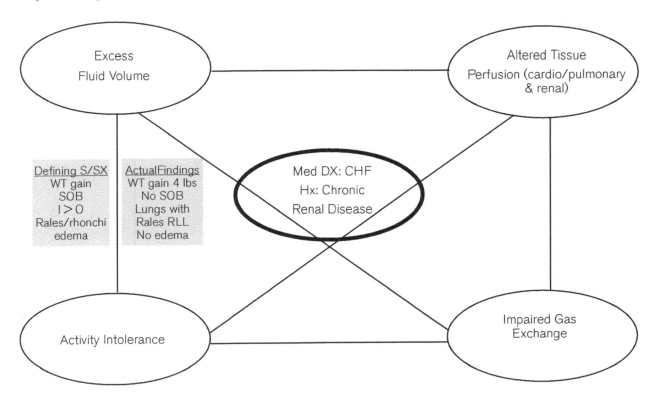

assessing for edema on this CHF client. The monitoring, comparing, contrasting, and trending of the clinical assessment findings leads to early identification and/or prevention of potential complications. This is an expected and essential competency required of a new graduate nurse that directly impacts the safety of the client.

Learning Point: After reviewing the prior data you have assessed, you want to make sure you have identified the priority clinical assessment findings for the nursing diagnosis of Excess Fluid Volume. If, for example, you left out daily weight as a priority clinical assessment finding, remember monitoring daily weights is the best method of determining fluid status in a client.

Assuming in this case you have included the priority clinical assessment findings, ask yourself the following inquiry questions:

1. *"What clinical findings indicate that your client may have excess fluid volume?"*

2. If you stated the client gained 4 lbs., ask yourself, *"Is this a weight gain over the past week or in the past 24 hours?"*

Let's assume for learning purposes, that you did not know. Your next question to yourself would be:

3. *"Why would this be important to know if your client gained or lost weight in the past 24 hours?"*

Using these inquiry questions, you are developing your clinical reasoning skills to recognize that a 4 lb. weight gain in 24 hours is a significant clinical finding and helps validate excess fluid volume. Repeat this process for all of the nursing diagnoses on the concept map.

STEP 5: Determine Outcomes and Evaluation Criteria

Setting outcomes are very difficult for students because you have so little experience. This makes it difficult to do outcome-focused thinking. Here is an easy way to help yourself learn how to develop outcomes. Transform the nursing diagnosis into a positive term. For example, let's take the diagnosis, "Excess fluid volume" and ask, "What is the positive of this problem?" The answer is "Fluid Volume Balance". . . voilà the **OUTCOME**!

The next step is to determine if the outcome was met and if so, how do you know that? You develop evaluation criteria using the same process where you used the assessment data and transform them into desired outcomes. For example, one of the assessments for excess fluid volume is "weight gain of 4 lbs since yesterday". The desired outcome can be measured by the evaluation criterion of "weight gain < 2 lbs per day.

The following table illustrates the outcome and evaluation criteria development process for all of the client problem/nursing diagnoses used in this example.

Determine Outcomes and Evaluation Criteria Table

Client Problem/ Nursing Diagnosis	Clinical Assessment Findings	Outcome	Evaluation Criteria
Excess fluid volume	• Weight gain 4 lbs from yesterday • Lungs with rales in left lower lobe • c/o SOB	Fluid Volume Balance	• Wt gain < 2 lbs/day • Lungs clear • No SOB • No edema
Activity Intolerance	• Increase SOB • Increase pulse from 85 to 96 BPM with activity • Pulse returns to baseline 10 min after activity	Tolerates Activity	• No SOB • Pulse within client's norm • Pulse returns to baseline < 3 min after activity
Impaired Gas Exchange	• c/o of SOB • c/o of anxiety • Respirations 23/minute • O_2 Sat 91%	Adequate Gas Exchange	• No SOB • No c/o of anxiety • Respirations 16–20/min • O_2 Sat > 95%
Altered tissue perfusion	• Capillary refill > 3 sec • Pulses + 1 • Skin cool • Color pale	Adequate tissue perfusion	• Capillary refill < 3 sec • Pulses +2 • Skin warm and dry • Color pink

STEP 6: Interventions

Now that the outcomes have been established, we can move forward with the interventions that will help achieve the outcomes. It is very important to select the best interventions to achieve the outcomes using the compare and contrast thinking strategy (Chapter 3). Using the same example client in the concept, the table below illustrates this process with the four nursing diagnoses used.

Client Problem/ Nursing Diagnosis	Clinical Assessment Findings	Outcomes	Evaluation Criteria	Interventions
Excess fluid volume	• Weight gain 4 lbs from yesterday • Lungs with rales in left lower lobe • c/o SOB • No edema	Fluid Volume Balance	• Wt gain < 2 lbs /day • Lungs clear • No SOB • No edema	• Weigh daily, compare & trend • Assess I & O • *Assess Lung sounds* • *Cough and deep breathe q 4 hrs* • *Incentive spirometer every hour while awake* • *Semi-Fowler's position* • *Assess SOB* • *Assess edema*
Activity Intolerance	• Increase SOB • Increase pulse from 85 to 96 BPM with activity • Pulse returns to baseline 10 min after activity	Tolerates Activity	• No SOB • Heart rate within client's norm • Ht rate returns to baseline < 3 min after activity	• *Assess SOB* • Teach client to pace activity • Assess pulse and RR before, during and after activity
Impaired Gas Exchange	• c/o of SOB • Lungs with rales in left lower lobe • Respirations 23/min • O_2 Sat 91%	Adequate Gas Exchange	• No SOB • Lungs clear • Respirations 16-20/min • O_2 Sat > 95%	• *Assess SOB* • Assess for restlessness • Assess RR and O_2 sat • Administer O_2 as ordered • *Assess lung sounds* • *Cough and deep breathe q 4 hrs* • *Incentive spirometer every hour while awake* • *Semi-Fowler's position*

Developing Outcomes and Evaluation Criteria With Interventions (cont'd)

Client Problem/ Nursing Diagnosis	Clinical Assessment Findings	Outcomes	Evaluation Criteria	Interventions
Altered tissue perfusion	• Capillary refill > 3 sec • Pulses + 1 • Skin cool • Color pale	Adequate tissue perfusion	• Capillary refill < 3 sec • Pulses +2 • Skin warm and dry • Color pink	• Assess cap-refill q 4 hrs • Assess pulses, color and skin temp q 4 hrs • Position with legs uncrossed • *Legs level with heart* • *Semi-Fowler's position*

Developing Outcomes and Evaluation Criteria With Interventions

The next phase in this process is to determine the priority interventions for the client. The nursing interventions in bold print in the chart above are priority because they help achieve more than one client outcome. The other interventions are distinct to that particular nursing diagnosis and outcome. When you see all of the interventions on a concept map; you are better able to determine which interventions will be most effective for the most outcomes. This exercise helps you to do system thinking and to see the whole client picture versus looking at each client problem/ nursing diagnoses and outcome separately.

Learning Point: Using inquiry and reflection questions can help you understand why a particular intervention would help achieve the outcome. For example, the assessment finding of rales and rhonchi in the left lower lobe indicates that you need an intervention every four hours to assess the lung sounds.

1. *"What intervention would help clear fluid from the lungs?"* This question will lead you to the intervention of deep breathing and coughing and incentive spirometer.

2. *"What position would best help the client to breathe easier?"* This question would guide you to the intervention of positioning in Semi-Fowler's.

As you progress during the semester, increase the complexity of the inquiry questions you ask yourself. For example, *"What medications are the clients taking that will assist in achieving the outcomes?"*

STEP 7: Evaluation and Clinical Judgment

The next step is to determine if outcomes have been achieved. This is not a yes or no answer, but a process of comparing the evaluation criteria to the client's current clinical findings. There are three clinical judgments that are possible.

✦ Outcome met

✦ Outcome partially met

✦ Outcome not met

Now that a decision about outcome achievement must be made, you have to decide what you are going to do next. What are your nursing responsibilities? This is clinical judgment. Clinical judgment uses a series of reflective questions to help make a clinical judgment about future client care as indicated in the questions below.

OUTCOME NOT MET

1. Did the client's situation change (i.e., the client had a respiratory arrest)?
   a. If yes, revise plan of care to correspond to the new client condition.
   b. If no, go on to the next question.
2. Were the interventions ineffective?
   a. If yes, revise the interventions.
   b. If no, go on to the next question.
3. Did I evaluate too soon or is more time needed for the interventions to be effective?
   a. If yes, continue the current care and continue to evaluate.
   b. If no, go to next question.
4. Were the conclusions drawn from the clinical assessment findings accurate?
   a. If yes, continue the current plan of care and continue to evaluate.
   b. If no, re-analyze the clinical assessment findings to determine correct client nursing diagnosis and outcome, and revise the plan of care.

OUTCOME PARTIALLY ACHIEVED

If the outcome was partially achieved, then you would use similar reflection questions.

1. Is more time needed for the interventions to be effective?
    a. If yes, continue the current plan of care and continue to evaluate.
    b. If no, go to next question.
2. Are changes needed in the interventions to achieve the outcome?
    a. If yes, make the changes. Increase frequency of the interventions or add new interventions.
    b. If no, continue plan of care and ongoing evaluation.

OUTCOME ACHIEVED

1. Is the problem likely to recur without nursing interventions?
    a. If no, discontinue nursing diagnosis.
    b. If yes, go to next question.
2. Does the nursing diagnosis require the same level of intervention or vigilance?
    a. If yes, continue plan of care.
    b. If no, revise plan of care to meet current needs of client.

It is common for students to say, "The client does not have this nursing diagnosis because they have no signs and symptoms, so I need to take it off the concept map."

It is very important that you understand there is high risk of reoccurrence of excess fluid volume in a client with CHF and renal failure. *It would not be safe practice to quit monitoring for the clinical findings of fluid volume excess when the problem is likely to reoccur.* The prudent nurse will monitor for potential complications. Therefore, excess fluid volume would remain on the concept map. Here are two examples of inquiry questions to help guide you in this judgment process:

1. *"Your client has CHF with renal failure; what is the risk that excess fluid volume may occur?"*
2. *"What would you want to continue to monitor to prevent complications?"*

STEP 8: Documentation

Following judgment, you will need to document in the chart your conclusions. The concept map is a useful guide for you while documenting. It is important that documentation contain the following three pieces of information:

+ Client's response to interventions

+ Progress toward the outcomes

+ Any changes in plan of care

The concept map and your clinical recording sheet (see Chapter 3) should provide all of the information you need to document accurately.

PUT THE CONCEPT MAP INTO CLINICAL PRACTICE

The development of the concept map begins when you receive your clinical assignments. If you are not able to assess your assigned client before clinical, you can still begin the concept map using the prototype case (see Chapter 3). The concept map may change after you actually assess your client. The table on page 41 describes how the clinical instructor helps you put the concept map into clinical practice. The chart also describes how your clinical instructor will be helping you use the concept map in clinical practice.

Putting the Concept Map into Clinical Practice

Student Responsibility	Clinical Instructor Responsibility	Teaching Points
1. Hypothesize potential nursing problems/nursing diagnoses around the assigned client medical diagnosis(es)and bring concept map to clinical.	• Review concept map at the beginning of clinical. • You may want the students to complete separate patho, lab and med and student clinical recording sheets while they are learning (see Chapter 3).	• Does the concept map reflect the prototype client for this diagnosis(es)? If so, go to number 3. • *Remember that the concept map will not have individualized care at this point.* • *If the concept map does not reflect appropriate hypotheses, then this is a teaching opportunity to guide the student, go to number 2*
2. If hypothesized concepts are incorrect after speaking with the clinical instructor, then edit or add to the concept map. *Hint: Use pencil initially to complete concept map. Use different color pencils for different diagnoses.* DO NOT ERASE; just put an X through the revision or change colors, so you can see the CHANGE in THINKING and LEARN from this. Do not start over!	• Guide the student to include concepts that would be part of prototype client. • After the assessment, the student can cross through what was not appropriate and add what they found. • Instruct the students not to erase and start over. Using this process, you can see the change in the student's thinking.	• *(Expectation of what student should have done will be based on level of student.)* • Important to remind students that what they did the night before was not a waste of time, but a learning process to make judgments based on their assessments and the plan of care is constantly evolving to meet the needs of the client.
3. Assess your client and revise concept map as appropriate.	• Re-evaluate the concept map as the student makes changes. • (This may be done orally during the clinical day, depending on the level of the student.)	• If student was on the right track with the concept map, but after the assessment of the client revisions were needed, it is the responsibility of the clinical instructor to help the student realize this is part of the process.

Interaction between you and your clinical instructor is similar as you work through each of remaining steps 3 through 7 in constructing the concept map.

The concept map is an established best practice for teaching you clinical reasoning. Using the concept map does require practice and repetition. When used in each clinical, the concept map becomes an internalized part of your thinking. As you progress in your learning, you will be able to transition from the written concept map to oral presentations of the concept map in your last semesters of school. Systematic thinking, once illustrated through a written concept map, becomes a critical thinking habit you will use in your clinical practice.

At the end of this chapter for your reference and use are an **Example of an Outcome Concept Map**, **Criteria for Grading the Outcome Map** (both of which can also be used with nursing diagnoses or outcomes), and a **blank Nursing Diagnosis and/or Concept Map** for you to use (pages 43-46). In addition, other clinical forms that we have found helpful and that can be adapted to your needs are included: **AIDES, Medication Information Form for students, Client History and Pathophysiology Information Sheet, Health History and System-Specific Assessment Tool,** and a **Lab, Diagnostic Tests, and Procedure Recording Form** (pages 48–54).

EXAMPLE OF OUTCOME CONCEPT MAP

Name _____   Clinical Faculty _____   Sec # _____   Date _____   Grade _____

Nursing Diagnosis: Ineffective breathing patterns

Outcome: Client will achieve optimal respiratory function

System-Specific Assess	Outcome Desired	Interventions
1. c/o of SOB	1. No SOB	1. HOB↑
2. RR– 26	2. RR 16–20	2. C & DB q 4 hrs
3. Rales LL bilaterally	3. Lungs clear	3. O_2 @ 2L NC
4. O_2 Sat > 95%	4. O_2 Sat > 95%	4. O_2 Sat q 4 hrs/note changes
		5. Auscultate lungs q 4 hrs

Nursing Diagnosis: Activity Intolerance

Outcome: Client will improve and/or maintain activity tolerance

System-Specific Assess	Outcome Desired	Interventions
1. RR & P ↑ with activity	1. RR & P return to norm within 3 min of activity	1. Monitor RR & P before and after activity
2. c/o of SOB with activity	2. No SOB with activity	2. Teach pursed-lip breathing with activity
3. Not pacing activity	3. Pace activity	3. Teach to prioritize and pace activity
4.	4.	4.

Medical DX
CHF

and Pertinent History
Diabetes

Nursing Diagnosis: Knowledge Deficit of Low Na Diet

Outcome: Client will know how to maintain a Low Na Diet

System-Specific Assess	Outcome Desired	Interventions
1.	1.	1.
2.	2.	2.
3.	3.	3.
4.	4.	4.

Nursing Diagnosis: Excess fluid Balance

Outcome: Client will maintain fluid balance

System-Specific Assess	Outcome Desired	Interventions
1. Wt gain 5 lbs/24 hrs	1. Wt within 2 lbs of norm	1. Daily wt & compare
2. I = 1240 cc > O	2. I = O	2. Monitor I & O q 8 hrs
3. Rales LL bilaterally	3. Lungs clear/no SOB	3. O_2 @ 2L NC
4. 2+edema bilaterally in LL legs	4. ↓ to no edema	4. Legs position lower than heart ROM or walking
		5. Monitor edema q 4 hrs & compare

EXAMPLE OF OUTCOME CONCEPT MAP, PAGE 2

Name_____

1. Outcome: Client will achieve optimal respiratory function
Client response to interventions:
1. HOB ↑, Pt stated ↓SOB and was able to breath without labor
2. O_2 2 l/cannula cont, O_2 sat 98%
3. Lungs Rales↓ in R lobe, remain in Llower lobe
Clinical Judgment: Was overall outcome met   Yes_____   Partially x_____   Not at all_____

Why (Rationale, explain your judgment): What would you do differently?

Continue current interventions. Saw improvement in adventitious lung sounds, but still has productive cough and rales remain in Left lower lobes. Positioning and O_2 decreased SOB and Increase O_2 Sat.

2. Outcome: Client will maintain fluid balance
Client response to interventions:
1.
2.
3.
4.
Clinical Judgment: Was overall outcome met?   Yes_____   Partially x_____   Not at all_____

Why (Rationale, explain your judgment): What would you do differently?

3. Outcome: Client will improve and/or maintain activity tolerance
Client response to interventions:
1.
2.
3.
4.
Clinical Judgment: Was overall outcome met?   Yes_____   Partially x_____   Not at all_____

Why (Rationale, explain your judgment): What would you do differently?

PRIORITY LAB/PROCEDURES	RESULTS/INTERPRETATIONS	NURSING INDICATIONS (PRE & POST)
1. Electrolytes, NA & K	Na – 138mEq/L K – 3.2mEq/L	Notify Dr. prior to giving Lasix because of low K
2. Blood Sugar, HbA1c	HbA1c – 7%	Continue insulin as ordered/monitor for effect
3. BUN/Creat	BUN 19/ Creat 1.9	Continue to monitor because of CHF, diabetes and receiving ace inhibitor

EXAMPLE OF CRITERIA FOR OUTCOME CONCEPT MAP

Student Name _____   Clinical Instructor _____   Date _____   Grade _____

Directions: Complete one **Nursing Outcome Concept Map** each week. You will get a Pass/Fail. One of the written outcome concept maps will be graded and one will be presented orally to your clinical instructor on designated weeks. The average of the two will be 5% of your application grade. You will receive your assigned client and primary medical diagnosis(es) when you arrive for clinical. Get the client report, do your assessment and then do the first page of the outcome concept map. The outcome concept map is a working tool, so **make appropriate changes/additions through the day as the clinical situation dictates. Use a different color ink or pencil color to make changes in the concept map.** You are to complete the first page of your concept map by the end of the clinical and your clinical instructor will review and sign. The final review will be completed when all components of the concept map, 2 medication AIDES sheets and reflection page are turned in/emailed to your faculty. SBAR will be given according to resource on blackboard or per unit protocol.

CONCEPT MAP COMPONENTS WITH CRITERIA FOR GRADING	POINTS EARNED/ POINTS POSSIBLE PASS/FAIL	CONCEPT MAP COMPONENTS WITH CRITERIA FOR GRADING	POINTS EARNED/ POINTS POSSIBLE PASS/FAIL
1. Based on the patient's medial diagnoses, draw a nursing outcome concept map **using 3 priority outcomes,** one of which should be a teaching and discharge outcome. *2 points for each of the three outcomes that are a priority 2 x 3 = 6*	____/6 ____P/F	6. **State if outcomes were met and make a judgment about each outcome based on your evaluation** (i.e., continue, modify, discontinue) and why. *2 points for each outcome judgment x 3 = 6*	____/6 ____P/F
2. Identify at least **4 measurable assessments and assessment findings for each outcome.** Write them under the appropriate outcome on the concept map. *2 points for each assessment and assessment finding, 8 points per outcome x 3 outcomes = 24*	____/24 ____P/F	7. **Interpreted correctly 3 priority lab values** related to the patient's current clinical conditions with **nursing indications.** *2 points per each correctly interpreted lab value and nursing indications x 3 = 6*	____/6 ____P/F
3. Identify at least **3 priority nursing interventions that will help achieve each outcome.** Write them beside the assessment findings under the nursing outcome concept map. **Note: Must include at least 2 action interventions** (i.e., cough & deep breathe every 2 hours **and 2 priority assessments for monitoring** the client's response (i.e., monitor VS every 4 hours and compare to previous finding). *1 point per intervention per outcome if appropriate & meet criteria*	____/12 ____P/F	8. **Describe 2 medications and identify nursing indications and expected client response for each of the three medications.** *3 points for each medication (1 point for indication and 2 points for expected response) 2 x 3 = 6*	____/6 ____P/F
4. Use lines to show the relationships between the outcomes. Different colored pencils for each outcome to draw the lines can make the relationships clearer. *Points based on relationships being valid*	____/6 ____P/F	9. **Critical Thinking/Reflection Questions** are answered completely and clearly with appropriate detail. **See Reflection page.** *12 available points*	____/12 ____P/F
5. On second page of concept map clearly **evaluate the client's response to each of the interventions and progress toward meeting outcomes.** *1 point for each of the evaluation responses for the intervention.* *4 points/outcome x 3 = 12*	____/12 ____P/F 100	10. **Correctly prepare and give SBAR report to clinical instructor prior to reporting off to the assigned RN.** *10 points possible*	____/10 ____P/F 100
Total Points Possible			**Total Points Received**

Handout 3

NURSING DIAGNOSIS AND/OR OUTCOME CONCEPT MAP TOOL

Name _____ Clinical Instructor _____ Sec # _____ Date _____ Grade _____

Medical Dx and Pertinent Hx

Nursing Diagnosis:

Outcome:

System-Specific Assess	Outcome Desired	Interventions
1.	1.	1.
2.	2.	2.
3.	3.	3.
4.	4.	4.

Nursing Diagnosis:

Outcome:

System-Specific Assess	Outcome Desired	Interventions
1.	1.	1.
2.	2.	2.
3.	3.	3.
4.	4.	4.

Nursing Diagnosis:

Outcome:

System-Specific Assess	Outcome Desired	Interventions
1.	1.	1.
2.	2.	2.
3.	3.	3.
4.	4.	4.

Nursing Diagnosis:

Outcome:

System-Specific Assess	Outcome Desired	Interventions
1.	1.	1.
2.	2.	2.
3.	3.	3.
4.	4.	4.

Reviewed day of clinical by: Clinical Instructor signature: _____ Date_____

NURSING DIAGNOSIS AND/OR OUTCOME CONCEPT MAP TOOL, PAGE 2

Name _____

1. Outcome:

Patient response to interventions:

1.

2.

3.

4

Clinical Judgment: Was overall outcome met?   Yes _____   Partially _____   Not at all _____

Why (Rationale, explain your judgment): What would you do differently?

2. Outcome:

Patient response to interventions:

1.

2.

3.

4.

Clinical Judgment: Was overall outcome met?   Yes _____   Partially _____   Not at all _____

Why (Rationale, explain your judgment): What would you do differently?

PRIORITY LAB/PROCEDURES   RESULTS/INTERPRETATIONS   NURSING INDICATIONS (PRE & POST)

1.

2.

3.

AIDES MEDICATION INFORMATION FORM

Directions: Please complete on _____ of your priority medications

Turn into clinical instructor _____

Have ready as information for all drugs you are administering (book, drug cards)

"AIDES" to Assist in Remembering Facts for Medication Administration

Name of Drug: Brand_____ **Generic**_____

Classification_____

A Action of medication:

Administration of medication. Dosage ordered_____

How to administer:

Assessment:

Adverse Effects. List significant ones:

Accuracy/Appropriateness of order. Is it indicated based on client's condition, known allergies, drug-drug or drug-food interactions? If not, what action did you take?

I Interactions (Drug-Drug, Food-Drug):

Identify priority plan prior to giving drug (i.e., vital signs, labs, allergies, etc.):

Identify priority plan after giving drug:

D Desired outcomes of the drug:

Discharge teaching—Administration considerations for client and family:

E Evaluate signs and symptoms of complications. Intervene if necessary and describe:

S Safety (client identification, risk for falls, vital sign assessments):

REFERENCE:

HISTORY AND PATHOPHYSIOLOGY INFORMATION

Student Name _____ Faculty _____Sec #_____

Date _____   Pass/Fail or Grade_____

Directions: Complete and email to clinical instructor by _____.
(10 points possible on graded web noted on Rubic for Outcome web)

Client's Story (History)—What brought him/her to the hospital?

PATHOPHYSIOLOGY

Please describe the etiology (cause) and pathophysiology in your words. This is to be completed for the major diagnosis and any other active diagnoses that affect care (i.e., diabetes).

List the signs and symptoms of the disease from the textbook. Compare it to the clinical system specific assessment findings from your client (may complete the comparison after you care for your client during clinical).

Assessment findings (signs & symptoms)   Assessment findings my client manifested:
from textbook:

_____   _____

_____   _____

_____   _____

_____   _____

_____   _____

_____   _____

_____   _____

Handout 6

HEALTH HISTORY AND SYSTEM-SPECIFIC ASSESSMENT TOOL

Demographic Information	
Source of History	
Chief Concern/Complaint	
History of Present Illness (HPI)	
Past Medical History (PMH)	
Family History (FH)	
Social History (SH)	
Health Promotion Behaviors	
Review of Systems (ROS) System-Specific as indicated by client condition: • Integument • Head and Neck • Eyes • Ears, Nose, Mouth and Throat • Breasts • Respiratory • Cardiovascular • Gastrointestinal • Genitourinary • Musculoskeletal • Neurological • Mental Health • Endocrine • Allergic/Immunologic	
Focused History of Symptom • Location • Quality • Quantity • Timing • Setting • Alleviating or Aggravating Factors • Associated Phenomenon	

II PHYSICAL ASSESSMENT

General Survey
1. Appearance
2. Level of Consciousness
3. Behavior/Affect
4. Posture/dress
5. Signs of discomfort or distress
6. Assess pupils for symmetry, shape, reactivity light

Skin Assessment:
1. Color
2. Condition—Look behind ears, skin folds, between toes, soles of feet, pressure areas on shoulder, sacrum, heels
   Presence or absence or lesions, scars, wounds or piercings
3. Texture
4. Temperature
5. Skin turgor sternum
6. Nails condition, presence of clubbing
7. Capillary refill bilaterally fingers

Respiratory Assessment
1. Rate
2. Rhythm
3. Accessory muscle use
4. Chest shape and symmetry/spinal deformities/AP: LA
5. Ausculation 12 sites anterior, posterior and axillary—assess for presence or absence of adventitious sounds, cough, congestion

Cardiac assessment
1. PMI—assess location and size
2. 4 auscultation sites with diaphragm and bell
   a. Aortic—2nd RICS RSB
   b. Pulmonic—2nd LICS LSB
   c. Tricuspid—4th LICS, along left lateral sternal border
   d. Mitral or apical pulse—5th LICS MCL, apex of heart
3. Carotids—assess pulse quality, presence or absence of thrills/bruits, bilaterally
4. JVD
5. Lymph

Abdomen
1. Size
2. Shape
3. Symmetry
4. Condition—presence or absence of piercings, scars, striae, pulsations, peristalsis or bulges
5. Bowel sounds—assess all 4 quads, # sounds per minute RLQ
6. Assess for distention or tenderness with light palpation

Extremities
1. Capillary refill to UE
2. Assess UE and LE for general range of motion
3. Assess UE and LE for condition, color, temperature and presence of edema
4. Palpation of peripheral pulses—radial and dorsal pedalis
5. Assess clonus

Handout 7

LAB & DIAGNOSTIC TESTS AND PROCEDURES FORM

Use as Weekly Reference

Name: _____

Date: _____

Client Initials: _____

Directions: Identify all pertinent labs to the client condition, whether normal or abnormal. Describe what caused the client to have an abnormal lab or why a lab may now be normal (e.g., norm WBC–client on antibiotics). Also explain why you would or would not call the MD about this lab. These laboratory values may vary in textbooks. Look at the accepted norms for the institution where the test is interpreted to determine abnormal versus normal. This list is not all inclusive.

Lab Test	Date of Lab Test	Results	Normal	Pertinence to Client	Would You Call the MD?
Hematology					
WBC			$5.0 - 10.0 \ 10^3$ ul		
RBC			$4.2 - 5.4 \ 10^6$ µL		
HGB			12.0 – 16.0 g/dL		
HbA1c			7% or less		
HCT			37.0 – 47.0%		
MCV			$81 - 89 \ \mu m^3$		
MCH			26 – 35 pg/cell		
MCHC			31 – 37 g/dl		
Platelets			150,000– 400,000/mm³		
Neutrophils			37 – 75%		
Lymphocytes			19 – 48%		
Monocytes			0 – 10%		
Eosinophils			1 – 3%		
Basophils			0.0 – 1.5%		
Chemistry					
Sodium			135 – 145 mEq/L		
Potassium			3.5 – 5 mEq/L		
Chloride			98 – 107 mEq/L		
Glucose–serum			70 – 110 mg/dL		
Magnesium			1.3 – 2.1 mEq/L		
BUN			6 – 20 mg/dL		
Creatinine			0.7 – 1.4 mg/dL		
Calcium			9.0 –10.5 mg/dL		
Protein			6.0 – 8.0 mg/dL		
Albumin			3.5 – 5.0 mg/dL		
A/G Ratio			1.5:1.0 – 2.5 :1.0		
Total Bilirubin			0.3 –1.3 mg/dL		
Direct bilirubin			0 – 0.4 mg/dL		
Indirect Bilirubin			0.2 – .8 mg/dL		
ALT, SGPT			10 – 30 U/L		
AST, SGOT			8 – 46 U/L		

Lab Test	Date of Lab Test	Results	Normal	Pertinence to Client	Would You Call the MD?
LDH – serum			91 – 180 mg/dL		
Alk Phos			35 – 142 U/L		
Uric Acid			2 – 7 mg/dL		
Phosphorus			2.5 – 4.5 mg/dL		
Total Cholesterol			< 200 mg/dL		
LDL age > 45 (LD)			90 – 185 mg/dL		
HDL			40 – 65 mg/dL		
Triglyceride			35 – 150 mg/dL		
Urinalysis					
Color			Clear Yellow		
Appearance			Clear		
Glucose			Neg.		
Bilirubin			Neg		
Ketones			Neg		
Specific Gravity			1.015 – 1.025		
Blood			Neg		
Ph			5 – 9		
Protein			Neg		
Urobilinogen			0.5 – 4.0 mg/24hr		
Nitrates			Neg		
ABG's					
pH			7.35 – 7.45		
pCO_2			35 – 45 mm Hg		
pO_2			80 – 100 mm Hg		
HCO_3			22 – 26 mEq /L		
O_2 Sat			> 95%		
Type of O_2 client receiving					
Digoxin			0.5 – 2.0 µg/ml		
Dilantin			10 – 20 µg/ml		
Tegretol			4 – 12 µg/ml		
Theophylline			10 – 20 µg/ml		
Pt			12 – 14 SEC		
Ptt			30 – 45 SEC		
Amylase			25 – 125 U/dL		
Cardiac Enzymes					
Myoglobin			30 – 90 ng/ml		
Total CPK			Male 5 – 55 U/L		
(CK)			Female 5 – 25 U/L		
CPK-MB			0 – 7% of total CPK		
CPK-BB			0% of total CPK		
CPK-MM			5 – 70% of total CPK		
Troponin I Value			< 0.6 ng/ml		
BNP			< 100 pg/ml		

DIAGNOSTIC TESTS/PROCEDURES

1. X-Ray, Endoscopy, Scans, Biopsy, C & S, or other special procedure reports

    Test: _____

    Date: _____

Conclusion/Interpretations: _____

    _____

    _____

Pertinence to Client: _____

2. X-Ray, Endoscopy, Scans, Biopsy, C&S, or other special procedure reports

    Test: _____

    Date: _____

Conclusion/Interpretations: _____

    _____

    _____

Pertinence to Client: _____

3. X-Ray, Endoscopy, Scans, Biopsy, C & S, or other special procedure reports

    Test: _____

    Date: _____

Conclusion/Interpretations: _____

    _____

    _____

Pertinence to Client: _____

CHAPTER 5

Interactive Strategies for Clinical

IN THIS CHAPTER YOU WILL:

→ Explore methods to create a positive clinical learning environment

→ Examine interactive strategies

While clinical can be anxiety-producing to both you and your clinical instructor, it can also be fun. Remember the word **GAME** to help you and your clinical instructor discover some fun and effective learning strategies.

G – Group and Team Work

A – Active Learning

M – Meaningful Partnerships

E – Eliminate Passive Learning

G - GROUP AND TEAM WORK

Today's generation of students see learning as social activity and feel it should be fun as well. Clinical provides an optimal opportunity to capitalize on team work. Working in pairs is a very effective way to help the novice clinical student gain confidence as you rely on each other's strengths and knowledge. Learning how to build cohesive teams in clinical is very important as peer support is a major variable in positive job satisfaction and patient safety when you enter the work force.

A – ACTIVE LEARNING

The most effective way to learn is through the active engagement with the content. This is true of both knowledge and psychomotor skills. Although today's students are skilled in accessing information instantly through the internet, you may have limited ability to distinguish what is reliable versus unreliable. In clinical, your instructor's role is to create an environment where you must find the information independently and make decisions about how that information would be applied in clinical. During clinical, it is an expectation that you will learn how to acquire needed information, a competency required in the professional nurse. Clinical is the perfect place for this to occur.

M – MEANINGFUL PARTNERSHIPS

Students today thrive in an environment where they have a meaningful partnership with their clinical instructor. There is an extensive discussion of strategies you can use to develop successful learning partnerships in Chapter 6.

E – ELIMINATE PASSIVE LEARNING

Clinical is an active learning environment. You are responsible for seeking opportunities for additional learning while you are in clinical. For example, if you know that a client needs a nasogastric tube inserted, take the initiative to ask if you can do this skill, even if it is not your client. Some ways your clinical instructor may engage you is through simulation scenarios, case studies, and stories of real-life experiences. For example, your clinical instructors may post case studies that require you and your fellow students to edit or add nursing interventions specific to the client-scenario using wiki software. This could be an ongoing case study in real-time, incorporating new clinical information and skills learned in clinical or in the classroom. This provides an excellent opportunity to connect the nursing concepts learned in the classroom to clinical learning and requires you to be fully engaged. The interactive clinical teaching strategies listed below are examples of ones we have used and know will increase active learning. Review these and see if there are any you might want to share with your clinical instructor.

Interactive Clinical Strategies

Game	Description	Use
Scavenger Hunt	• Work in groups of 2 or 3 • Locate items on a unit and describe their exact location • Each group will take the others to the location	• Helpful during clinical orientation to identify location of essential equipment, supplies
Skill Day	• A planned clinical day for clinical skill review	• Can use early each semester to review new, previously learned and/or practice clinical skills
Clinical Scene Investigation—CSI	• Identify a mystery, unknown clinical fact, and/or dilemma such as "why is the patient suddenly itching?" • Generate a list of possible explanations, such as drug-drug interactions, allergy, contact dermatitis, etc. • Investigate the different explanations until you arrive at a conclusion, or realize you do not have enough data to solve the mystery	• Helps you seek out needed information • Also helpful for group learning • (Hint: This is a great strategy when you do not know the answer!)
Deck of Doom	• Card Game that reviews a clinical situation on a card • Each student should take a card • You have to answer and report back to the group at post-conference • An example may include the following: The client's blood sugar at 1 PM is 47 mg/dL; what are the priority nursing interventions for this client?	• Post conference game, or to be used for fun during the clinical day • Use to reinforce learning, such as hard-to-remember concepts, like the onset, peak times of different insulins • Use in the classroom for new information or test review
Leading Learning for the Day	• Ask your clinical instructor if you can be paired with another student to assist with clinical learning or serve as a leader for a student team	• Helpful confidence builder • Helps develop leadership, teambuilding and collaboration skills • Helpful to use when the clinical situation is very busy • Beneficial exercise during senior semesters

Interactive Clinical Strategies (cont'd)

Game	Description	Use
War Stories	• Clinical instructors or students share clinical experiences that can be positive or negative or even funny • Who can tell the best story?	• Connections between reality-based practice with theoretical learning • Stories are a vivid personal learning method that students can connect with • Stories may involve both positive and negative clinical experiences • Ice breaker for a new clinical group • Bonding experience among clinical group and clinical instructors • A reflection exercise for the end of the semester
Who Wants to be a Millionaire?	• Note: Ask your clinical instructor if you can play "Who Wants to be a Millionaire?" Here are the instructions: • They can answer the question themselves • They can ask another student (call a friend) • They can ask the group (poll the audience) and choose to agree or disagree with the answer	• This is a great strategy to reduce the tension • Reinforce content while still holding the students accountable for their learning • For example, can be used prior to medication administration, procedures, post conference and/or the classroom

CHAPTER 6

Collaborating With Multi-Generational Learners

> ## IN THIS CHAPTER YOU WILL LEARN ABOUT:
>
> → Traditionalists and Baby Boomers as clinical instructors
>
> → Characteristics of Generations X and Y students
>
> → Learning strategies for Generations X and Y

When you combine the characteristics of a novice learner (Chapter 1) with the characteristics of Generations X and Y, it is apparent that there are differences in attitudes, values and learning styles. Often, the majority of clinical instructors are Baby Boomers, with a few Traditionalists and Generation Xs, but the majority of our students are Generations X and Y (Millennial). It is important to understand that you and your clinical instructor may have differences in the way you learn and teach. Open communication is critical to maximize your learning. This means you need to let your clinical instructor know when you do not understand or need the information presented in a different way. The discussion below illustrates these differences.

TRADITIONALISTS AND BABY BOOMERS AS CLINICAL INSTRUCTORS

There are challenges and opportunities for clinical instructors and students who are Baby Boomers. First of all, Baby Boomers have had to learn new technology and accept that tried and true ways do not always work. It is hard to adapt to less-is-more in communicating with Generations X and Y.

CHARACTERISTICS OF GENERATIONS X AND Y STUDENTS

Generations X and Y are culturally diverse. They want balance in life; they like informality and to have fun; are highly independent and good problem solvers, but ironically require frequent feedback. They have been raised with high expectations, for example that nothing less than an A is acceptable. This can lead to frustration during the learning process. The Generations X and Y students want to know why they need to learn "this?" They do not want extraneous material, they just prefer concrete, specific information. Generations X and Y desire personal interaction with the clinical instructor and want to be a partner in the learning process.

They are technologically literate, creative, and grew up multi-tasking . . . talking on the cell phone while working on the computer, and doing their homework. However, it is impossible to think about more than one thing at a time. In fact, what the students in these two generations do is toggle back and forth between the subjects. The danger is students then have difficulty learning anything in depth. It is a challenge for clinical instructors to turn off the toggle switch in their students and help them do outcome focused thinking.

STRATEGIES FOR GENERATIONS X AND Y

There are important strategies that students can use in developing partnerships with their clinical instructor. If you are a Generation X or Y student, some strategies using the word **COACH**, can help you successfully work together.

C – **Collaborate and Create Partnerships**

O – **Off with the Toggle Switch**

A – **Acquire the Knowledge**

C – **Communication**

H – **Have to Solicit Frequent Feedback**

C – COLLABORATE AND CREATE PARTNERSHIPS

As a clinical student you can help contribute to a positive learning environment. Learning occurs best in an environment where the student feels safe and there is mutual respect. This environment can be created by treating everyone equitably and with respect, speaking in a calm, controlled voice, and turning in clinical papers when due. There are many other ways, but all of these help establish a trusting partnership between you and your clinical instructor.

Generations X and Y respect the clinical instructor as an expert, but they want to partner with their instructors in the learning process. It is still the responsibility of the clinical instructor to set expectations and adhere to standards of practice and safety. As students, you expect to be respected as learners and want to be included in the decisions about your learning. Your role in the partnership means that you assist in making decisions, participate in your own learning and ask questions in a collaborative manner. Challenging the clinical instructor in a negative way is not beneficial to the partnership and does not contribute to your learning. Strong interpersonal skills are essential for successful partnerships.

O – OFF WITH THE TOGGLE SWITCH

Generations X and Y students are adept with multi-tasking, however multi-tasking is the toggling between one activity to another at a very rapid pace. Generations X and Y's ability to be on the cell phone, texting, and "Googling" information—all while they are doing their concept map—is impressive. Their ability to access large amounts of information is a great skill to have, but unfortunately this can be overwhelming. Your clinical instructor is a valuable resource to help you prioritize what is important. With so many distracters competing for your attention, strategies for turning off the "toggle switch" and focusing on one topic in depth is imperative. Strategies introduced in chapters 2 and 3 that can help are:

+ Know what is expected of you

+ Use established structures, such as the Medication Protocol

+ Be prepared for clinical

+ Know that repetition is critical for learning

+ Learn from inquiry and reflection questions

+ Use thinking strategies

These strategies will encourage critical thinking beyond the knowledge level to develop the clinical reasoning skills that will be required of you as a new graduate nurse.

A – ACQUIRE THE KNOWLEDGE

Critical thinking and clinical reasoning are the desired outcomes for students in clinical. However, you cannot think about nothing, so it is essential that you acquire the base knowledge that you need. Knowledge acquisition begins in the classroom, but the true learning occurs when it is applied in clinical. One of your responsibilities as a student is to bring the knowledge you learned in the classroom to clinical. This is observed through your ability to construct a concept map, skill in assessing, nursing interventions, medication administration, procedures, and following healthcare provider orders.

While you are very familiar with technology, such as computers and smart phones, you have used this technology primarily for social networking. Now you need to learn how to use this technology to acquire essential knowledge needed to provide safe and effective care that is based on good critical thinking and clinical decision making that achieves desired outcomes. The use of smart phones in clinical and the availability of eBooks allow you to have instant access to needed information. Your clinical instructors will help you learn how to seek current, evidence-based information, such as CINAHL or MEDLINE.

C –COMMUNICATION

Generations X and Y tend to communicate cryptically because of extensive time spent on electronic communication. Although emailing, instant messaging, and now tweeting and twittering, with family, friends, and people from different countries through the Internet have become common practice; that is very different than the therapeutic communication required for client care. This can be as simple as how to address different generations, for example, the need to address traditionalists formally with Mr. or Ms. or Sir; to being able to relate informally with Generations X and Y clients. Knowledge of interpersonal as well as therapeutic communication skills by you will make a significant difference in your ability to establish rapport with clients and the healthcare team.

Strategies to help you improve your communication skills are very important. Here are some suggestions to use during clinical:

+ Interactive role-playing and practice in lab

+ Interpretation of non-verbal client behaviors

+ Role modeling appropriate therapeutic communication

+ Feedback about your interactions with clients

+ Simulation scenarios on effective communication

Communication is an essential skill, best learned in clinical, that impacts the therapeutic relationships that you have with your clients, and is a major factor in patient safety.

H – HOW TO SOLICIT FREQUENT FEEDBACK

Generations X and Y are at home in a technological world. They grew up with interactive computer games, Nintendo, X-Box and Wii, and expect immediate feedback about how they are doing. Unlike Traditionalists and Baby Boomers, these two generations expect feedback on a frequent basis. Without frequent feedback, students have difficulty proceeding in the learning process or will incorrectly assume they are right. If your clinical instructor is a Baby Boomer, it is very easy for there to be a difference in perception between your clinical instructor and you about your performance. If you are a Generation X or Y student, you may perceive the information to mean you just need to make a few changes. However, your clinical instructor means this is not correct or acceptable, and you need to change your behaviors immediately. Generations X and Y need explicit feedback on exactly what needs to happen. Because it is important not to leave the feedback open to interpretation, it is your responsibility to seek clarification about the meaning of the feedback you receive. It is very important for you and your clinical instructors to discuss when you can expect to receive feedback throughout your clinical.

NOTES

CHAPTER 7

Assessment and Evaluation

IN THIS CHAPTER YOU WILL LEARN ABOUT:

→ Criteria for clinical evaluation

→ Using feedback effectively

→ Participating in the evaluation process

One of the most anxiety producing aspects of being a student is the clinical evaluation process. Your clinical instructor has the responsibility of judging whether you are able to give safe and effective care at your current level and are ready to move forward to the next semester or to graduation. This is a huge responsibility. In this chapter we will describe the process of clinical evaluation.

Evaluation is the ongoing process of observing, measuring, and judging students' progress toward achievement of clinical performance outcomes. Students need to know what evaluation criteria will be used and what the consequences will be if they do not meet the criteria. Effective evaluation will:

✦ Improve skills and abilities

✦ Motivate student development

✦ Achieve student outcomes

ESTABLISHING CRITERIA FOR CLINICAL EVALUATION

The first step is to determine expectations and clinical outcomes. The course syllabus must define the expected student clinical outcomes with clear measurable evaluation criteria. There are two levels of evaluation that are ongoing in clinical evaluation. These decisions about evaluation criteria are established by your faculty team and are outlined in the syllabus or the student handbook. As students, you are held accountable for this information.

Another area in which you will be evaluated is student behaviors that violate patient safety standards. Your syllabus will define what constitutes unsafe care practices. These will include but are not limited to:

+ Failure to follow the 7 Rights of Medication Administration

+ The number and nature of medication errors that will be allowed as part of the learning process

+ Failure to follow infection control standards

+ Failure to follow patient safety standards

+ Failure to adhere to HIPAA laws

+ Failure to report important clinical information in a timely manner to the clinical instructor or nursing staff

+ Failure to document nursing assessments, interventions, evaluation of care

+ Performing nursing actions without supervision when supervision is required

+ Any nursing action or event that could result in harm or death of a client

Criteria will also include expectations for attendance, tardiness, and professional attire. Other clinical expectations as outlined in Chapter 2 also serve as guidelines for evaluation.

USING FEEDBACK EFFECTIVELY

Feedback provides students information on their strengths and weaknesses. The more timely the feedback, the more powerful it is. Feedback helps to define for students the expectations on what they need to do each week to meet the clinical performance outcomes.

The fear of receiving feedback in clinical is shared by many students. It is difficult to hear negative feedback about clinical performance. What you may perceive as negative feedback from your clinical instructor, is constructive feedback intended to help you improve your clinical performance. Avoid being defensive and be open to the information your clinical instructor is giving you. Reflect on the feedback, ask questions for clarification and develop a plan for improvement.

Here are some important elements about the feedback you receive. It should:

+ Be specific about behaviors observed

+ Describe who, what, when, where and how

+ Be timely

+ Give in private; never in front of others

+ Use "I" statements to relate your reactions

The following "Pitfalls" illustrate what NOT to do when receiving performance evaluation feedback from your clinical instructor.

+ Avoiding feedback
  Pitfall: You will have no idea if you are doing well or not well

+ Negative body language like rolling your eyes or sighing
  Pitfall: The message is disrespectful and conveys a negative attitude

+ The Snapback—responding immediately without thinking in a harsh tone
  Pitfall: It makes you appear intimidated and out of control

+ Defensive statements
  Pitfall: Blocks effective communication and growth

Feedback is also ineffective and unacceptable when you express yourself in highly emotional terms or make dire predictions like, "I might as well just quit nursing school" or "I am never going to pass this clinical."

Feedback often requires judgment by the clinical instructor. Here are two examples of a student failing to meet the expectation of being prepared for clinical that have two different outcomes. Read the examples and see why they had different outcomes. Which student do you want to be? We hope you chose the second student. In this example, the student took the initiative to meet the requirements for clinical.

EXPECTATION IS STUDENTS COME PREPARED FOR CLINICAL

Example 1:

> A student comes unprepared to clinical and states, "I was unable to find the information on my medications I am to give today."
>
> *Instructor Action*: The student should be sent home and given a clinical day failure.
>
> *Rationale*: This constitutes an unsafe care environment for the client and the student failed to meet a basic expectation for clinical.

Example 2:

> Student says, "I was unable to find the information on my drugs I am to give today. I looked in my medication book and searched the web. This morning I plan to call pharmacy to get the information on the drug."
>
> *Instructor Action*: Give positive feedback
>
> *Rationale*: The student's action represents information searching and problem solving, both excellent critical thinking attributes.

PARTICIPATING IN THE EVALUATION PROCESS

The concept map provides a valuable tool for you to use in clinical and provides your clinical instructor information about your thinking. What you write on your concept map is an external representation of your thinking. The most important aspect of the concept map is that you can see the progression of your thinking and the development of your clinical judgment. The concept map is an evolving document that changes as client conditions change and as you improve your ability to provide appropriate care and make clinical judgments in both clinical and simulation experience. The handout, **Helpful Tips When Doing Simulation**, on page 76 will help you be prepared for both clinical and simulation.

Below are ways your clinical instructor may use the concept map as an evaluation tool.

+ The value of requiring a concept map before clinical is to assure you are safe and are prepared for clinical.

+ The emphasis on evaluation and/or grading the concept map is placed on your ability to make changes based on your assessment of the client, the client's response to the care, and evaluation and judgment about the care given.

Your clinical instructor knows you are becoming more sophisticated in your clinical reasoning when you are able to evaluate and use clinical judgment to make decisions about what care is needed in the future. An example of the criteria that can be used to grade the concept map can be found at the end of Chapter 4.

As we stated earlier, evaluation is an ongoing process. Clinical instructors are looking for trends in your clinical performance. Weekly evaluations are done to identify trends and to give you timely feedback. The advantages of weekly evaluations are that they provide:

+ Trends: positive or negative

+ Documentation

+ Timely feedback

+ Motivate student development

+ Assist clinical instructors with clinical assignments

The purpose of the evaluation tool is to define the clinical outcomes the faculty have determined are necessary to meet clinical objectives. The evaluation criteria measure what you are expected to achieve. The **Example Evaluation Tool** included at the end of the chapter reflects criteria that you may be evaluated on, such as the nursing process, patient safety standards, clinical application of key NCLEX® standards, professional behaviors, and required written clinical care plans or concept maps. The course syllabus will state the process for clinical evaluation to include when counseling is necessary and what constitutes clinical day failures and when the clinical day failures result in course failure.

As you review the example evaluation tool, ask yourself, "What can I do to demonstrate what I am learning to my clinical instructor?" This is a great question considering that most of the time there is one clinical instructor and at least 8 students! Here are some suggestions:

+ Wow your instructor by being prepared (Refer to "**SAFETY Format**" **Study Guide** on page 77)

+ Keep your clinical instructor informed about what you are doing

+ Impress your clinical instructor with your thorough nursing documentation (Refer to **Example of Nursing Documentation** on page 78)

+ Demonstrate you know how to give an SBAR report (See handout on page 79)

+ Write about what you have learned in your reflection paper or journal

+ Share your contributions in post conference

+ Take the initiative to find new learning experiences

Weekly evaluation provides you the necessary information about your progress. Below are some questions your clinical instructor will use to evaluate your weekly progress. This is where the trends become evident.

+ Is the student receiving "satisfactory" every week and making acceptable progress?

+ Is the student receiving some "needs improvement" in certain areas but you observe progress in the area the next week?

Clinical Instructor Action: None needed, continue to evaluate and document student's progress

But:

+ Is the student receiving "needs improvement or unsatisfactory" in the same areas over a number of weeks with no progress?

Action: Counseling session needed.

Counseling serves to notify you formally that your performance is unsatisfactory. There are two levels of counseling that your instructor may use:

+ The counseling session identifies needed actions or behaviors to progress and includes consequences if they do not improve.

+ The counseling session identifies a significant event or action that resulted in, or potentially could have resulted in, patient harm and the ensuing consequences, i.e., clinical day failure or course failure.

A common structure for counseling is the "STAR" format. This is a concise format, easy to use and keeps both clinical instructors and students focused on the facts of the situation. (See **Unsatisfactory Course Performance Clinical Day Failure** on page 80.)

STAR FORMAT FOR COUNSELING

S = Situation: Describe the situation

T = Task: What was supposed to be accomplished, or what were the requirements, standards of practice or policies that were not met? Include standards or policies as appropriate.

A = Action: Plan for Action: What does the student need to do to improve?

Consequences: What are the consequences if corrective action is not taken? A time frame for improvement must be stated.

R = Results: Follow-up sessions: Were actions accomplished? What was the outcome?

If it is decided that a counseling session is necessary, here is what may occur:

✦ You will be informed that your clinical instructor is concerned about your clinical performance, and you will be notified when the counseling session will occur.

✦ A counseling form such as the "STAR" format will describe the situation with specific information.

✦ Most likely the course coordinator or other neutral party will witness the counseling session.

✦ You will be notifiued of the scheduled counseling time.

✦ The structure of the counseling session will include: purpose of the meeting, introduction of the witness, and begin with discussion of the situation as written on the counseling form.

✦ You need to be prepared to stay on the topic that is being discussed. Now is not the time to bring up other issues.

✦ Although it may be very difficult, try not to become emotional. Ask for a moment to excuse yourself if you need to control your emotions.

✦ After the clinical instructor has presented the situation, you will be given an opportunity to express your side of the story. (Note: there is usually a place on the form for you to write your comments.)

✦ After you present your side of the story, actions and consequences will be discussed.

✦ At the conclusion of the session, you will be asked to sign the form. Your signature only indicates you have seen the form and the session occurred. You can write in the comment section if you disagree.

✦ You will be given a copy of the counseling statement.

✦ REMAIN CALM AT ALL TIMES!!!!!!

It does not matter when an unsafe event occurs. If it was unsafe on the first day of clinical, it is unsafe on the last day of clinical.

Most of the time, the evaluation process is positive. The purpose of the evaluation process is to help you improve your skills and abilities, and motivate you for future growth and best of all, be successful in achieving the clinical outcomes.

CLINICAL EVALUATION TOOL

CLINICAL EVALUATION TOOL

Student Name:																																								
Clinical Date:																																								
PERFORMANCE OUTCOMES	S	NI	U	NA	S	NI	U	NA	S	NI	U	NA	S	NI	U	NA	S	NI	U	NA	S	NI	U	NA	S	NI	U	NA	S	NI	U	NA	S	NI	U	NA	S	NI	U	NA
Prepared for all facets of clinical day (skills, drugs, patho, etc.)																																								
Assessment																																								
Performs system-specific assessments; i.e., physiology, psychosocial, culture, spiritual																																								
Recognizes deviations from client's normal																																								
Analysis: Nursing Diag. Concepts, Outcomes																																								
Formulates appropriate nursing dx, concepts, desired outcomes using assessment																																								
Planning																																								
Identifies specific, measureable outcome criteria																																								
Develops interventions to obtain desired outcomes																																								
Implement Interventions																																								
Implement priority nursing interventions																																								
Perform nursing procedures with supervision as needed																																								
Med protocol (preparation/ administration/ documentation)																																								
Discuss appropriate principles of delegation, room assignment for specific client's needs																																								
Notifies instructor/ nurse (trends /changes in client condition, complications with meds and/or post procedure) & intervene as appropriate																																								
Evaluation																																								
Evaluation of progress toward desired outcomes																																								
Evaluate medications for desired outcomes, undesirable effects, interactions																																								

CLINICAL EVALUATION TOOL (cont'd)

CLINICAL EVALUATION TOOL

Student Name:

Clinical Date:

The evaluation grid uses repeated rating columns: **S | NI | U | NA** across multiple clinical dates.

PERFORMANCE OUTCOMES

Clinical Judgement
- Assess if progress toward outcomes is being met; makes changes as appropriate

Safety/Infection Control
- Seeks guidance when appropriate
- Maintains client safety (fall prevention, bed position, call light, infection control, equipment, etc.)

Communication
- Written communication/ charting is complete, timely and cosigned by end of shift
- Oral Communication: uses theraupeutic communication techniques
- Non-verbal communication: Aware of importance & impact of non-verbal behavior
- Gives concise, accurate, compete report at end of day following SBAR before leaving
- Pt teaching concise, accurate; includes health promotion & plan for transitional care

Professional Behavior
- Integrates standards of care, scope of practice & ethical practice into client care
- Coordinates/colloborates/advocates with interdisciplinary team
- Accepts constructive criticism
- Maintains client / institutional confidentiality; i.e., HIPAA
- Assertive in seeking learning experiences

Page 2

CLINICAL EVALUATION TOOL (cont'd)

CLINICAL EVALUATION TOOL

Student Name:

Clinical Date:

PERFORMANCE OUTCOMES	S	NI	U	NA	S	NI	U	NA	S	NI	U	NA	S	NI	U	NA	S	NI	U	NA	S	NI	U	NA	S	NI	U	NA	S	NI	U	NA
Respectful of all patients/personnel																																
Reports on time to unit/conferences & utilizes spare time constructively																																
Follows dress code																																
Outcome Web																																
Written /Oral Outcome web 1st page completed, with priority interventions identified based on assessment, evaluation of pt response & progress toward outcomes																																
Paperwork turned in on time																																
Faculty/student initials																																

S: Satisfactory; NI: Needs Improvement; U: Unsatisfactory; NA: Not experienced

S: Clinical behavior is safe & demonstrates growth toward course competencies

NI: Clinical behavior is safe; however, performance is deficient in essential background knowledge

U: Clinical behavior is unsafe. Performance seldom demonstrates essential knowledge & growth toward competencies

NA: Clinical behavior not relevant to assigned patient

Absences:_____   Late arrivals:_____

Final Clinical Grade:_____

Faculty:_____   Date:_____

Student:_____   Date:_____

Comments:

Page 3

Handout 2

HELPFUL TIPS WHEN DOING SIMULATION

REQUIRED EQUIPMENT

▲ Stethoscope

▲ Penlight

▲ Scissors

▲ Pen/paper (clipboard)

▲ Watch with a second hand

PROFESSIONAL APPEARANCE

▲ Hair in compliance with clinical dress code

▲ Proper uniform with name tag

▲ Fingernails clean and short

▲ Minimal jewelry

TEAMWORK

T Team player; no one person is in charge unless specifically assigned by the faculty member.

E Each student should actively participate (i.e., check orders, prepare meds, check IV site and fluids, communicate with the client, etc.).

A All assessments, observations, communications and tasks should be communicated **out loud** to facilitate group decision making and give faculty insight into your thinking/planning process.

M Must divide up activities, prior to starting the scenario, that need to be done and revise these weekly (i.e., if student A does vital signs one week; student B will do them the next).

S Speak up if you feel you are not on the right track or another student is about to perform an unsafe/inappropriate action, don't back down! Talk it out with your team.

FUNCTIONAL POINTS

O Orders from the Health Care Provider and medication record are available at bedside.

R Review the location the supplies are kept for the scenario.

D Decide if lab results need to be requested and request to have them available. If none are available the facilitator will state as much.

E Evaluate and know the method for calling the HCP or other ancillary personnel.

R Real client . . . Treat mannequin as a real client and ask them questions and respond to their comments and questions.

REMEMBER THAT ACTIVITIES YOU DO IN THE HOSPITAL WHEN ENTERING THE CLIENT'S ROOM ARE ALSO EXPECTATIONS DURING SIMULATION (i.e., handwashing, identifying self using first and last name and your role as an RN, and identifying client using two identifiers).

Remember you signed a Confidentiality Agreement to maintain scenario integrity. Sharing information devalues student experiences, skews evaluation and/or grading expectations against earlier teams, and decreases learning experience for later teams.

"SAFETY FORMAT" STUDY GUIDE

Components of SAFETY	**S**ystem Specific Physiology, Etiology, Assessment	**A**nalysis of Assessment	**F**irst do Priority Interventions	**E**valuation of Expected Outcome	**T**rend, Potential Complications	**Y**es to Management To Prevent RISK and Yes to Questions
Explanation of SAFETY Components	How does the disease pathology relate to the clinical manifestations? What are risk factors for the condition? What signs or symptoms are the patient exhibiting that indicate the disease process is taking place? What lab values or diagnostic tests results need to be evaluated? What findings should be reported to the provider? What assessments may indicate development of a potential complication?	What nursing diagnoses or nursing concepts are relevant to the client's assessment and disease pathology?	What are the priority nursing interventions that will help improve the assessments noted in the analysis of assessment? What are priority physician / provider's orders that need to be implemented? What medications are ordered for administration? What immediate interventions are necessary when a complication develops?	How did the interventions affect the client? What changes in the client assessment are expected to result from the interventions performed? What evaluation assessments indicate the interventions were successful? Was progress made toward the expected outcome? Given the client response, what revisions should be made to the plan of care? What is the expected outcome of the medications ordered?	What baseline assessments are "normal" for the client? How does the current assessment differ from the initial admission assessment? How does the current assessment compare to assessment performed on the previous shift? Have there been any changes noted in assessment findings? What assessment findings can indicate a trend? (i.e, VS, I&O, LOC, pain, tube drainage, etc.—ALL!!)	What is the Standard of Care? What findings are priorities to report to the healthcare provider? Are the client's orders appropriate for the assessment and disease process? What activities or tasks can be delegated to another RN, LPN, or UAP? What teaching points are needed by the client? Is this client at RISK for: • Falls • Infection • Equipment

Handout 4

EXAMPLE OF NURSING DOCUMENTATION

0800	Admission Note: Admitted 75-year-old African American male with a history of stable COPD x 2 years, Hypertension, and right sided CVA from the clinic. Complains of fatigue, increasing cough and shortness of breath (SOB) over past 3-4 days. A week ago, began waking up in the middle of the night with acute SOB, and for the last three nights, has been unable to sleep. Complains of chest pain with an excessive cough that is productive. Admission chest x-ray reveals right middle lobe pneumonia. States has been a smoker x 40 years; reports drinking 3 or more alcoholic beverages daily. Denies allergies. Alert, oriented to person, place and time (A&O x3), with coherent thoughts, PERRL. Vital signs on admission: BP-140/90 L arm sitting, Apical pulse-110 bpm, Resp-32/min, Temp-102.4° F, Ht-5' 9", Wt-223 lbs , Pulse Ox-92%, O_2 via nasal cannula (NC) at 2 liters. Monitor shows sinus tachycardia. No S_3 or S_4 on auscultation. Uses accessory muscles for breathing, dyspnea on exertion, chest slightly barreled. Expiratory wheezes present with wet crackles in lung bases bilaterally, complains of chest pain when coughing. Cough productive with thick yellow green sputum. Lips - slightly cyanotic and is using pursed lip breathing. Client reports unable to sleep for 3 nights, needs an extra pillow and has abnormal fatigue and weakness. Skin cool; dry, intact with no lesions, bruising, urticaria, petechiae, rashes or ecchymosis. Cap refill > 3secs, moderate clubbing and cyanosis. Jugular vein distention (JVD) w/ HOB @ 30 degrees present. All peripheral pulses equal and regular. Abdomen slightly distended, BS active x 20/min. Has active, full ROM. Currently has a TB skin test to his right forearm pending and is to be reassessed in 48-72 hours. Started on Moxifloxin IV, infusing in R hand.
0815	Raised head of bed to High-Fowler's, increase O_2 to 3L/NC, called Dr. Bill with client's SBAR report. (*Refer to SBAR report on next page*) Albuterol started via nebulizer treatment per order. Instructed client on the use of the incentive spirometer with return demonstration and how to do deep breathing and coughing (C & DB) every hour. Family at bedside.
0900	Client states he feels better. RR-25/min., O_2 sat 93%. O_2 decreased to 2 L per order. Monitor Sinus rhythm, HR-89 bpm. Has a productive cough with large amounts of thick yellow green sputum. Able to eat 1/3 of breakfast including eggs and toast.
1000	Client sleeping with HOB in High-Fowler's position family had bedside. Family is encouraging client to use incentive spirometer every hour.
1100	VS: Apical pulse-90 bpm, B/P-138/88, RR-25/min, O_2 sat-93%, Temp-101.5° F. Monitor showing sinus rhythm rate 85 bpm. Expiratory wheezes have decreased bilaterally. No other changes from previous assessment.
1200	Client able to get up to chair with assistance. Continues to experience SOB with exertion. Able to eat ½ lunch. Continue to have productive cough with large amounts of thick yellow green sputum.
1300	Assisted client back to bed. Position in High-Fowlers, P-105 bpm, RR-29., O_2 sat decreased to 90% with activity.
1315	Client P-92 bpm, RR-24/min, O_2 Sat-92% with O_2 2L/NC. Client states he is able to breathe easier. Completed nebulizer treatment per order.
1400	Report given to next shift. Client resting in bed, NSR per monitor, Heart rate-93 bpm, RR-24/min, O_2 continue 2L/NC. O_2 sat 92%. Crackles in lung bases diminished bilaterally from AM assessment. Continue with incentive spirometer and C & DB every hour. Continue to have productive cough with moderate amounts of thick yellow green sputum.

EXAMPLE OF A SBAR REPORT

(See explanation of SBAR Report on page 13)

S – SITUATION: Dr. Bill this is Carol, I am the nurse for Mr. Craig, age 75 in room 214 that you just admitted to the unit with right middle lobe pneumonia.

B – BACKGROUND: Mr. Craig has a history of COPD, HTN, and right sided weakness from a CVA five years ago. He has no known allergies

A – ASSESSMENT: I just completed the admission assessment and Mr. Craig is now in severe respiratory distress. His O_2 sats were 92% on admission, and are now 88%. I placed in him in High Fowler's, and adjusted his oxygen level to 3 liters per minute, and there has been no improvement. He has distended neck veins, cannot complete a sentence and is using accessory muscles to breathe. His BP: 150/92; Temperature: 98.6° F, HR 104 bpm; RR 32/min. He has inspiratory and expiratory wheezing bilaterally, and his wife states that he has used his bedside inhaler with no relief.

R – RECOMMENDATION: The nurse states: "I would recommend that a systemic bronchodilator (Albuterol, Proventil) via nebulizer treatment would be helpful as Mr. Craig uses this at home, but I need an order for it." What other orders Dr. Bill, do you recommend?" I am encouraging his use of the incentative spirometer and deep breathing and coughing exercises.

Handout 6

UNSATISFACTORY COURSE PERFORMANCE CLINICAL DAY FAILURE EXAMPLE STAR COUNSELING WARNING FORM

Faculty Name: _____   Student Name: _____

Date of Counseling Session: September 16, 2010   Date of Incident: September 10, 2010

S – SITUATION: Describe the situation. Course requirement not being met:

Gave Oxycodone, a narcotic, to her patient without the knowledge or supervision of the clinical faculty. (Reference: Number 6 under Medication Error Policy, page 10 of 323 Syllabus)

1. Could not answer questions about the actions of the medication. (Reference: Number 6 under Medication Error Policy, page 10 of 323 Syllabus)
2. Medication was not signed out, count was not done and no documentation of the medication was given. (Reference Number 5 under Medication Error Policy, page 10 of syllabus)
3. The patient was not assessed for level or type of pain. Patient's husband requested the pain medication for his wife. (Reference Number 5 under Medication Error Policy, page 10 of syllabus)

T – TASK: Requirements and/or policy performance standards that are not being met:

Reference: (Reference: Number 6 under Medication Error Policy, page 10 of Syllabus)

Student Medication Error Policy, page 10 of the Course Syllabus

Guidelines for clinical performance given in orientation for clinical on August 27, 2010

A – ACTIONS: to be taken to improve unsatisfactory performance:

1. All medications will be given under the supervision of your clinical faculty until you are notified otherwise.
2. Know the action and significant side effects of all medications prior to administering the medication.
3. All medications need to be correctly documented per hospital policy.
4. Failure to do so will result in a 2nd clinical day failure.

R – RESULTS: Date: Pending (Results from action listed above)

DATE TO IMPROVE PERFORMANCE BY: Immediately beginning with the next clinical day on Sept 17, 2010.

Faculty Signature: _____   Date: _____

Student Signature: _____   Date: _____

Observer Signature: _____   Date: _____

To be filed: Faculty files, Student file in Student Services

CHAPTER 8

Linking Clinical Experience to NCLEX® Success

IN THIS CHAPTER YOU WILL LEARN HOW TO:

→ Apply NCLEX® standards throughout the clinical experience

→ Adapt structures organized from the NCLEX® standards

APPLY NCLEX® STANDARDS THROUGHOUT THE CLINICAL EXPERIENCE

Clinical experiences are very important in preparing you for success on the NCLEX®. Now that you have reviewed the chapters in this book from how to start clinical through the evaluation process, let's move on to incorporating NCLEX® standards throughout the clinical experience.

Prior to linking clinical experience to NCLEX® success, it is important to begin with a review of some of the basic facts about the NCLEX-RN®. The purpose of the NCLEX-RN® is to ensure public protection. The exam evaluates specific competencies needed by the newly licensed, entry-level registered nurse to perform safely and effectively. The NCLEX-RN® Test Plan provides an abbreviated summary of the content and scope of the licensing examination. This plan is currently revised every three years. The Test Plan can be downloaded from the National Council State Board of Nursing's website (www.ncsbn.org). It provides a compass for preparation of the nursing student.

Linking these activities, as outlined in the NCLEX-RN® Test Plan, to the clinical experience is a very powerful strategy to ensure you have an appropriate focus during your clinical experience. For example, whether you are in medical-surgical, intensive care, obstetrics, or pediatric clinical, the NCLEX® Activity Statements will apply.

In order to prioritize these activities, we have adapted the mnemonics "**SAFETY**," "**RISK**," and "**AIDES**" to provide you with structures for organizing some of the NCLEX® activities. (Refer to Handouts 1, 2, and 3 on pages 86–88.)

ADAPT STRUCTURES ORGANIZED FROM THE NCLEX® STANDARDS

Some examples of how you may adapt the mnemonic "SAFETY" to linking the clinical experience to NCLEX® success begins with us starting to review the various letters beginning with the S in "SAFETY", "System-Specific Physiology." No matter what clinical rotation you are in, you must focus on understanding what is physiologically taking place with the client. In the beginning of clinical, it may be sufficient for you to understand the reason a school-age child is experiencing frequent swallowing after a tonsillectomy is due to bleeding. After you understand this physiological change, then you need to begin to understand the pathophysiology regarding the changes in the heart rate, respiratory rate, blood pressure, skin color and temperature, and urine output (if the bleeding is not evaluated and an early intervention is not implemented). This is a great opportunity for you to take advantage and compare these vital sign changes to different developmental stages. This will help you make the links and connections between adults and children. As you progress in clinical you will compare and contrast the similarities/differences in the physiology/pathophysiology between adults and children.

These two NCLEX® activities are essential to provide safe and effective care to your clients. You must be able to:

✔ Identify pathophysiology related to an acute or chronic condition (i.e., signs and symptoms).

✔ Assess and respond to changes in vital signs.

Another example of how clinical experience is linked to NCLEX® success is to review the S in "**Safety**" and "**System-Specific Assessment**." No matter what clinical rotation you are in, you need to reinforce and practice how to complete a fast system-specific assessment with a focus on the presenting symptoms. You have to learn to think "assess" from the minute you walk into the client's room. For example, if you are in the pediatric clinical rotation and the school-age child is bleeding after a tonsillectomy, then you need to connect that the unique system-specific assessment is the frequent swallowing and recognize the vital sign changes for the specific child. Then compare these vital sign changes to different developmental stages and/or even an adult. You can also connect the similarities and/or differences in both the system-specific assessments and the TRENDS with the hemodynamic changes that may occur with any client who is bleeding.

As you progress within the curriculum, it is important for you to review the differences between the system-specific assessments for a client who is bleeding post-op GI surgery, post cardiac catheterization, fracture, placenta previa, abruption placenta, etc. You must also learn to recognize the similarities between the hemodynamic changes that occur with any client who is bleeding. It goes without saying, that it is imperative to review the appropriate nursing interventions for the child who is bleeding following a tonsillectomy as well as comparing the differences/similarities in the nursing care for other clients who are bleeding for various reasons. With this process, you will have addressed four more NCLEX® activities.

✔ Perform focused assessment and re-assessment.

✔ Assess and respond to changes in vital signs.

✔ Recognize signs and symptoms of complications and intervene appropriately when providing care.

✔ Recognize trends and changes in client condition and intervene.

You also need to develop the habit of reviewing "**System-specific labs and diagnostic procedures**" through analyzing labs and performing diagnostic tests (i.e., EKG, O_2 saturation, glucose monitoring, etc.). During each clinical experience, you should review labs and link the significance of these to your client. In order to provide you with a structure for this, we have included a handout titled **Lab & Diagnostic Tests and Procedures Form** and a handout titled **Diagnostic Tests/Procedures** in Chapter 4. This process has addressed the following NCLEX® activities:

✔ Perform diagnostic testing.

✔ Evaluate the results of diagnostic testing and intervene as needed.

✔ Diagnostic Testing Assessment/Intervention.

✔ Lab values.

✔ Recognize signs and symptoms of complications and intervene appropriately when providing care.

The **A** in "SAFETY" stands for "**Analyzing priority nursing concepts.**" Now you review and assess several nursing needs for several different clients and prioritize the care for these clients. This is an excellent opportunity for you to learn how to appropriately triage or prioritize nursing care. This can also be a great topic for pre/post conferences. The NCLEX® activity addressed for this process is:

✔ Assess/triage clients to prioritize order of care delivery.

The **F** in "SAFETY" represents what nursing interventions should be implemented "**First**" as well as what medications should be administered first. When the client has 4 nursing interventions that need implemented, then you can ask yourself questions such as, *"What are the priority nursing actions?" "What medications should be administered first for specific clinical assessments?"* For example, if a client begins spitting out blood and the client is positioned in the supine position, then the first nursing action would be to reposition client even prior to notifying health care provider or initiating a complete assessment.

Here is another example of how you can prioritize. If the client has respiratory problems and has an order to administer a corticosteroid inhaler and a Beta$_2$ Adrenergic Agonist such as Albuterol, then you want to connect the actions for both of these drugs with the pathophysiology. This will assist you in understanding the rationale for administering Albuterol prior to the steroid inhaler. This brings us to the NCLEX® activity:

✔ Prioritize workload to manage time effectively.

The **E** in "**SAFETY**" will assist you to always remember to evaluate the "**Expected Outcomes**" from the nursing care as well as from the medications.

+ Did the bleeding stop?

+ Did the breath sounds improve?

+ Did the vital signs return to baseline?

+ Did the medication assist in reducing the intracranial pressure?

+ Did the medication assist in reducing the serum glucose?

The NCLEX® activities addressed include:

✔ Evaluate/document response to treatment.

✔ Evaluate therapeutic effect of medications.

"**Trends**" in the client's assessment, **T** in "SAFETY," is an excellent observation to determine if the client is stable. If client is not stable, then prioritize which nursing interventions need to be implemented immediately to prevent the client from experiencing a crisis. For example, if the client begins hemorrhaging two hours post-op, you need to assess the subtle changes with the heart rate and restlessness, and recognize the potential complication with bleeding prior to the client progressing to hypovolemic shock and intervene appropriately.

Another example of trends would be if the client was receiving Magnesium Sulfate and the urine output had been 85 cc/hour, and the next hour the urine output is 45 cc/hour. The Magnesium Sulfate is excreted in the urine, and with this trend it would be imperative to report this decline and not wait for the urine to continue to decline. You will need to learn how to think like this and it will take a lot of practice. With your clinical instructor's help, these clinical reasoning skills will become part of the structure for your thinking as you gain more clinical experience. This represents a new NCLEX® activity and requires thinking at the analysis level. The NCLEX® activities reviewed include:

✔ Recognize trends and changes in client condition and intervene.

✔ Recognize signs and symptoms of complications and intervene appropriately when providing care.

✔ Assess and respond to changes in vital signs.

The **Y** in "SAFETY" represents management. "**Yes, Management is important to prevent "RISK" to our clients!**" Refer to Handout 2 on page 87 for examples of NCLEX® activities reflecting Management and Safety on the NCLEX®. These activities will be useful for you to connect throughout clinical for both the client safety as well as to assist with NCLEX® success. From day one in clinical, you need to assess the following:

✦ Risk for falls

✦ Practice infection control (Refer to **Infection Control Procedures** on pages 89–90.)

✦ Identify client correctly

✦ Review accuracy of orders

✦ Assess and prevent skin breakdown

✦ Practice equipment safety

✦ Understand Standards of Practice

✦ Practice effective documentation

✦ Client teaching

The mnemonic "**AIDES**" is also a structure for organizing the NCLEX® activities that have a focus on pharmacology. This is a great tool to use throughout the curriculum, so you know what the expectations are from semester to semester. "AIDES" reflect NCLEX® standards, so if you consistently use this format, you will have a great understanding of what it takes to be successful on the NCLEX®.

These three mnemonics (pages 86-88) will serve as a compass to you while integrating NCLEX® standards during your clinical experience. Please note that while many of the NCLEX® activities from the NCLEX® Test Plan are represented throughout the mnemonics, these are not all inclusive. A complete list of these can be downloaded from the National Council of State Boards of Nursing (www.ncbn.org). It would be very powerful if from Day 1 in clinical you apply these standards in your clinical care and in your concept map. These standards also provide an excellent study guide to learn what is important to learn in the classroom as well. If you do this, you have provided yourself with an excellent roadmap to being successful on the NCLEX®. **The Quick Approach: Inquiry Questions for Clinical Knowledge Organized Around the Nursing Process** (Chapter 3) and the **Clinical Evaluation Tool** (Chapter 7) help link clinical to NCLEX®.

SAFETY

This structure can help prioritize NCLEX® activities that can be evaluated through the **Outcome Concept Map, History and Pathophysiology Information and Reflection Questions** (see Chapter 4 handouts).

S   System-specific physiology

system-specific assessment

system-specific labs and diagnostic procedures

A   Analyze priority nursing diagnoses/concepts

F   First do priority nursing intervention

First medications

E   Expected Outcomes

T   Trending changes and potential complications

Y   Yes, management is important to prevent "RISK" to our clients

Reference: National Council of State Boards of Nursing, Inc. (NCSBN) 2009

RISK

A structure for prioritizing Management and Safety NCLEX® Activities. Directions: *Please complete on your patient assignment. Turn into clinical instructor* _____.

R Room Assignments, Recognize limitations of staff, Restraint safety, Risk for falls, Receive or give report

I Identify trends, Infection control, Identification of client, Identify accuracy of orders, Informed consent

S Skin breakdown, Safe equipment, Scope of Practice for delegation

K Know Standards of Practice, Know how to document, Know how to teach

Reference: National Council of State Boards of Nursing, Inc. (NCSBN) 2009

AIDES

A structure for prioritizing Pharmacology NCLEX® Activities. Directions: *Please complete on ___ of your priority medications. Turn into clinical instructor* _____.

NAME OF DRUG: BRAND _____   GENERIC _____

CLASSIFICATION: _____

A   Action of medication:

Administration of medication. Dosage ordered_____

How to administer:

Assessment:

Adverse Effects. List significant ones:

Accuracy/Appropriateness of order. Is it indicated based on client's condition, known allergies, drug-drug or drug-food interactions? If not, what action did you take?

I   Interactions (Drug-Drug, Food-Drug):

Identify priority plan prior to giving drug (i.e., vital signs, labs, allergies, etc.):

Identify priority plan after giving drug:

D   Desired outcomes of the drug:

Discharge teaching—Administration considerations for client and family:

E   Evaluate signs and symptoms of complications. Intervene if necessary and describe:

S   Safety (client identification, risk for falls, vital sign assessments):

Reference: National Council of State Boards of Nursing, Inc. (NCSBN) 2009

INFECTION CONTROL PROCEDURES

STANDARD PRECAUTIONS

1. Wash hands immediately if they become contaminated with blood or body fluids.
2. Wash hands before and after client care and after removing gloves. Hand hygiene should be completed by using an alcohol-based waterless product and is recommended after contact with the client, body fluids, and contaminated equipment.
3. Wear gloves if you will or could come in contact with any body fluid, nonintact skin, mucous membranes and / or contaminated objects.
4. Gloves are removed and hand hygiene between each client.
5. Wear a gown, eye protection (goggles, glasses), or face shield, and a mask during procedures if likely to generate droplets of body fluids or blood.
6. Any client equipment that has been used handle carefully.
7. Implement hospital protocols for routine care, cleaning and disinfecting equipment, beds, bedrails, and environmental surfaces.
8. Contaminated laundry should be bagged and handled to prevent leaking or contamination of clothing or skin.
9. Needles or other sharp devices need to be handled carefully. Do not bend; break, place them into the original sheaths, or handle unnecessarily. Immediately discard after use into an impervious disposal box.
10. If the nurse has an exudative lesion, avoid direct client contact until lesion has been resolved.
11. A private room is not necessary unless client is unable or unwilling to maintain appropriate hygiene or contaminates the environment.
12. The specific substances covered by Standard Precautions include blood and body fluids, body secretions, and body excretions, except sweat, even with blood not being visible. Standard precautions also include nonintact skin and mucous membranes.

AIRBORNE TRANSMISSION–BASED PRECAUTIONS

1. Place client in a private room that has monitored negative air pressure (For fun and easy ways to remember additional facts about infection control refer to the book, *Nursing Made Insanely Easy*, Rayfield and Manning). The negative pressure airflow exchange in the room should have at least six exchanges per hours.
2. Both caregivers and visitors must wear masks or face shields when entering the room. These masks or respiratory protective devices should be an N95 or high-efficiency particulate air (HEPA) respirator if client is suspected to have tuberculosis.
3. Limit client transport out of room.
4. Clients who require this Airborne Precautions include (but not complete) measles, varicella, pulmonary or laryngeal tuberculosis, SARS.

INFECTION CONTROL PROCEDURES (cont'd)

DROPLET TRANSMISSION-BASED PRECAUTIONS:

1. Place client in a private room or with other clients with the same infectious disease.
2. When 3 feet of the client, wear a mask.
3. Keep visitors 3 feet from the infected client.
4. If client must leave the room, have client wear a surgical mask.
5. Clients who require Droplet precautions include (but not complete) meningococcal pneumonia/sepsis, mumps, mycoplasma pneumonia, pertussis, pneumonic plague, rubella, scarlet fever streptococcal pharyngitis or pneumonia.

CONTACT TRANSMISSION-BASED PRECAUTIONS

1. Place client in a private room or with other clients with the same infectious disease.
2. Wear gloves whenever the nurse enters the room. Always change gloves after contact with infected material. Prior to leaving the client's room, remove gloves and wash hands.
3. If clothing will have contact with client, surfaces in the environment, or client is incontinent of diarrhea wear a gown when entering the client's room.
4. Restrict movement out of the room for client.
5. Avoid sharing any equipment.
6. Disposal of infectious dressing material into a single, nonporous bag without touching the bag from the outside.
7. Clients who require Contact Precautions include (but not complete) gastrointestinal, respiratory, skin, or wound infections such as cellulitis, clostridim difficile, herpes simplex, major abscess, multidrug-resistant organisms, scabies, shigella.

TRANSPORTING THE CLIENT

1. Place a surgical mask on the client with an airborne or droplet infection and a draining wound is well covered if necessary to transport.

REPORTING COMMUNICABLE DISEASES

1. List of reportable diseases at CDC: (http://www.cdc.gov)

Bibliography

Asby, F.G. & Maddox, W.T. (2010). Human category learning 2.0., Annals NY Academy Science, December 2010.

Benner, P., Sutphen, M., Leonard, V., & Day, L. (2010). Educating nurses: A call for radical transformation. San Francisco: Jossey-Bass.

Benner, P., Tanner, C., & Chesla, C. (2008). Expertise in nursing practice. New York, NY: Springer Publishing Company, LLC.

Clark, C. (2008). Student perspectives on faculty incivility in nursing education: An application of the concept of rankism. *Nursing Outlook, 56,* 4-8.

Creech, C. (2008). Are we moving toward an expanded role for part-time faculty? *Nurse Educator, 33,* 31-34.

Dolan, G. (2003). Assessing student nurse clinical competency: Will we ever get it right? *Journal of Clinical Nursing,* 12, 132-141.

Gaberson, K.B. & Oermann, M.H. (2006). Clinical teaching strategies for nursing. New York, NY: Springer Publishing Company.

Herman, J., Manning, L., & Zager, L. (2011). The eight step approach to teaching clinical nursing. Duluth, GA: I CAN Publishing®, Inc.

Herman, J.W. (2008). Creative teaching strategies for the nurse educator. Philadelphia, PA: F.A. Davis.

Holden, C. (2009). Multitasking muddles the mind? http://news.sciencemag.org/ sciencenow/2009/08/25-02.html. Retrieved 12-1-2010.

Luhanga, F., Yonge, O.J., & Myrick, R. (2008). Failure to assign failing grades. *International Journal of Nursing Education Scholarship,* 5, 1-14.

Manning, L. & Rayfield, S. (2009). Pharmacology made insanely easy. Duluth, GA: I CAN Publishing®, Inc.

National Council of State Boards of Nursing. (2009). Report of findings from the 2008 RN practice analysis: Linking the NCLEX-RN® examination to practice. Chicago, IL.

Penn, B.K. (Ed.). (2008). Mastering the teaching role: A guide for nurse educators. Philadelphia, PA: F.A. Davis.

Pesut, D. & Herman, J.A. (1999). Clinical reasoning: The art and science of critical and creative thinking. Albany, NY: Delmar Publishing.

Rayfield, S. & Manning, L. (2009). Pathways of teaching nursing: Keeping it real! Duluth, GA: I CAN Publishing®, Inc.

Rayfield, S. & Manning, L. (2010). NCLEX-RN® 101: How to pass! Duluth, GA: I CAN Publishing®, Inc.

Skiba, D. & Barton, A. (2006). Adapting your teaching to accommodate the NET generation of learners. *The Online Journal of Issues in Nursing*. 11(2), Manuscript 4. Available: http://www.nursingworld.org/MainMenuCategories/ANAMarketplace/ANAPeriodicals/OJIN/Table of Contents/Volume112006/No2May06/tpc30_416076.aspx. Retrieved 12-15-2010.

Tanner, C. (2006). Thinking like a nurse: A research-based model of clinical judgment in Nursing. *Journal of Nursing Education*, 45, 204-211.

Zbat-Kan, E. & Stabler-Haas, S. (2009). Fast facts for the clinical nursing instructor: Clinical teaching in a nutshell. New York, NY: Springer Publishing Company.

Index

Other Books Published by I CAN Publishing®, Inc.

NCLEX-RN® 101: How to Pass!

NCLEX-PN® 101: How to Pass!

Nursing Made Insanely Easy!

Pharmacology Made Insanely Easy!

Pathways of Teaching Nursing: Keeping it Real!

The Eight-Step Approach to Teaching Clinical Nursing

★ ★ ★ ★ ★ ★ ★ ★ ★ ★ ★ ★ ★ ★ ★ ★ ★ ★ ★

CDs for Educators

Nursing Made Insanely Easy! Images on CD

Pharmacology Made Insanely Easy! CD review

★ ★ ★ ★ ★ ★ ★ ★ ★ ★ ★ ★ ★ ★ ★ ★ ★ ★ ★

I CAN Publishing®, Inc.
2650 Chattahoochee Drive, Suite 100
Duluth, GA 30097
866.428.5589
www.icanpublishing.com